THE TROUBLED

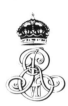

King Edward's Hospital Fund for London

Patron: Her Majesty The Queen

President: HRH The Prince of Wales

Treasurer: Robin Dent
Chairman of the Management Committee: The Hon Hugh Astor JP
Secretary: Robert J Maxwell JP PhD

King Edward's Hospital Fund for London is an independent foundation, established in 1897 and incorporated by Act of Parliament 1907, and is a registered charity. It seeks to encourage good practice and innovation in the management of health care by research, experiment and education, and by direct grants.

Appeals for these purposes continue to increase.

The Treasurer would welcome any new sources of money, in the form of donations, deeds of covenant or legacies, which would enable the Fund to augment its activities.

Requests for the annual report, which includes a financial statement, lists of all grants and other information, should be addressed to the Secretary, King Edward's Hospital Fund for London, 14 Palace Court, London W2 4HT.

BRYAN BROOKE

The troubled gut

THE CAUSES AND CONSEQUENCES OF DIARRHOEA

KING EDWARD'S HOSPITAL FUND FOR LONDON

Printed and bound in England by Hollen Street Press Ltd
Distributed for the King's Fund by Oxford University Press

ISBN 0 19 724635 4

King's Fund Publishing Office
2 St Andrew's Place
London NW1 4LB

Contents

Preface

Until recent times few knew or wished to know about scientific matters, particularly about medicine, except those directly involved through their work. Moreover lack of understanding about matters of health has been compounded by certain taboos. It is hardly more than twenty years since cancer began to be mentionable; it is still 'not done' to speak about death. Diarrhoea is very much under wraps, yet it is a condition that affects every one of us commonly in some way or other.

There are parts of the world so deprived of proper sanitation and hygiene that a normal bowel habit in the western sense is an unknown luxury. Even in our society, where hygiene usually prevails, breakdown does sometimes occur with devastating effects; more sinister is the undoubted increase of persistent diarrhoea. The way we live militates against a calm bowel; international travel adds to this dis-ease.

With better information the dire circumstances which afflicted individuals have to bear, and even epidemics, could be avoided, circumscribed or controlled. That alone is sufficient reason to break the taboo of silence surrounding the subject. There are other considerations. Up and coming people today have acquired a basis of scientific knowledge at school, and remain so orientated; medical matters are of interest, properly so, to our citizens. Today no society can be regarded as enlightened which lacks understanding of the way the body functions or the disorders which can disturb it. Furthermore in an age more sympathetic to the disabled than hitherto, wider cognisance of the effects of diarrhoea would bring comprehension, and thus more courtesy and concern to the unfortunate sufferers – all the more important because the incidence of chronic diarrhoea in at least one respect, Crohn's disease, is increasing.

To Dr Crohn and others I have turned for the genesis of my story. The nineteenth century saw the unravelling of the enteric fevers both as regards their identity and their cause; the symptoms and epidemiology of typhoid and dysentery were established, though how diarrhoea develops and how it can be overcome is very recent knowledge. The story of Dr Crohn marks the start of an epoch when, at the beginning of this century, chronic persistent diarrhoea not unlike dysentery began to plague us but with no obvious bacterial cause. We in this century have been less successful than the Victorians. By the middle of the last century they had identified the organisms responsible for typhoid and dysentery. This century is moving towards a close and we have yet to demonstrate any cause of our contemporary problem which has persisted since the time of Crohn and even before.

To tell the story of diarrhoea is easier said than done, for the mechanisms which bring this symptom in their train are complex and require an understanding of human biological mechanisms. The terms and concepts will present little difficulty to most readers; for those less fortunate in this respect I have endeavoured to make the meaning of unfamiliar words clear in the context in which they first appear.

Purists regard the appendage of a glossary as a sign if not admission of failure in a book of scientific bent for the uninitiated, on the grounds that the author should be able to make his meaning clear without such support. I subscribe to this view but make no apology for the Understanding of Terms, which will be found after the last chapter, for I am only too aware how difficult it can be as one gets older to take permanent hold of a new concept, word or term from a single exposure and explanation in a text. Since I have endeavoured to unfold the concepts stage by stage as they appear in the text, the Understanding of Terms may also prove helpful to those who wish to dip into the book at random.

PART ONE
The flux

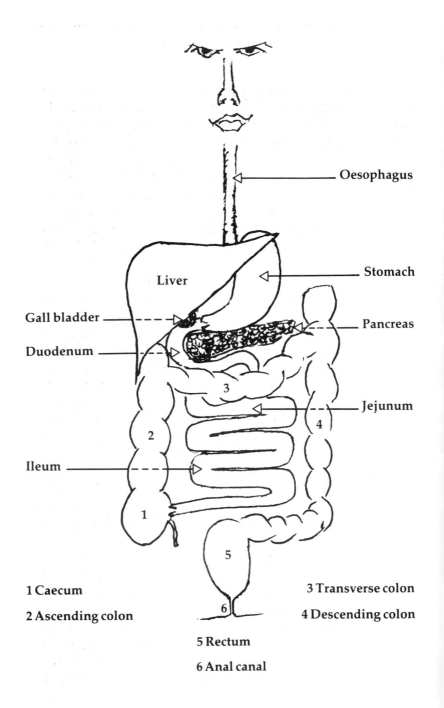

Oesophagus

Stomach

Liver

Gall bladder

Pancreas

Duodenum

Jejunum

Ileum

3

4

2

1

5

6

1 Caecum

2 Ascending colon

3 Transverse colon

4 Descending colon

5 Rectum

6 Anal canal

1 Dr Crohn and others

In 1932 New Orleans had not yet become the tourist attraction it is today with all the attendant disadvantages that entails. Street cars, trams as we call them, rattled up and down Canal Street as indeed they still did when I first saw the place a quarter of a century later and noticed one displaying as its destination the now famous 'Desire'. Today they are gone and the view down Canal Street towards the Mississippi is changed in many other ways: the most noticeable being a tower topped by a rotating restaurant, which quite eclipses the river boats moored below for trips down stream and back up the bayous – the canal systems which flank the river and keep the marshy lagoons drained. In the Vieux Carré, where I was able to eat two dozen oysters for tea at 32 cents a dozen, things have no doubt changed less, though the crumbling plaster on some of the buildings, including the famous mint julep bar, is not as old as it seems, being applied patchily for the 'vieux' effect. Strip-tease acts by girls on top of long bars to the rhythm of the jazz developed in the twenties and thirties continue today to the same beat, and will no doubt continue unchanged into the foreseeable future – just because New Orleans regards itself as the *fons et origo* of jazz.

In May 1932 something more sinister, and which was to prove more pervasive than jazz in the ensuing half century, was being described to a large gathering of doctors; it was the annual meeting of the American Medical Association. The speaker was a gastroenterologist. Gastroenterology, the study of illness affecting the stomach and intestines – anywhere from mouth to anus in fact – had only recently become a new speciality; previously such conditions had fallen within the ambit of general medicine and had come under the care of the general physician. But now a new breed of physician with a special interest had grown up within the USA though not yet in the UK – the gastroenterologist. In the early thirties, the gastroenterologist was more concerned with the stomach than the intestines if only because it was possible to study the stomach and what lay immediately next to it, the duodenum, more easily; he had x-rays at his disposal, and could take samples of gastric juice through a tube at 'test' meals. But the intestines were remote and hidden except at the further end, where a metal tube, originally made of lead, could be introduced into the rectum and through into the sigmoid colon just beyond, to obtain a direct view of the interior with the aid of light reflected into the sigmoidoscope, as this instrument is called, from a mirror. But that was too much like plumbing for many physicians who called in the surgeon to do the job – a menial task for a rather lower breed in their eyes, particularly so if he was a proctologist (proctology was then developing in the USA as a specialty confined to little more than the last inch and a half of the gut – a specialty which has never flourished in this restricted way in the UK).

The gastroenterologist on this occasion was a lively, aggressive and independent New Yorker with Jewish antecedents from Poland, Dr Burrill Crohn, rising 50 and that year the president of the American Gastroenterological Association; in 1920 he had become head of the department of gastroenterology founded in 1916 by a Dr Berg at Mount Sinai Hospital, New York. He was speaking about a condition new to his experience, and that of his colleagues, which caused diarrhoea in many patients, produced a mass to be felt on examination of the abdomen, and was found at operation to involve the region where small intestine ends and the large intestine begins – the ileocaecal area. Most important, this mass, which was not a cancerous growth, resulted from inflammation which when examined under the microscope revealed no special characteristics to identify its cause. In particular no tubercle bacilli could be demonstrated, an important negative finding since all cases with inflammation in the ileocaecal region had previously been thought to be tuberculous in origin.

The title of Crohn's paper was hardly felicitous – terminal ileitis. The 'terminal' referred not to the outcome however, but to the site of the disease in all the fourteen cases he was describing. On his return from the podium he sat down beside a gastroenterologist of some repute working at the Mayo Clinic; Dr Bargen shrewdly observed that it would be wiser to use the adjective 'regional' rather than 'terminal', for when more cases were seen the condition might be found to be located elsewhere in the ileum. And so it transpired. As in more recent times it has become evident that the condition may develop anywhere – in the mouth, stomach, gullet and onwards through the whole gut – so it has become difficult to retain an appropriate name based on its anatomical manifestations. Gradually the eponym 'Crohn's disease' has crept in as a convenient label, all the more so in that this keeps options open while the anatomical appellation tended to prevent consideration of the wider possibilities.

So the title Crohn's disease, gradually came about, the eponym starting in the UK and gaining currency during the last twenty years. Crohn's surgical colleague was the aforesaid Dr Berg. When Crohn proposed to Berg that they should collaborate in presenting a paper, the surgeon declined; he was too interested in collecting antique furniture and rare folios, and had no wish to be distracted from these absorbing pursuits in any way. So he let the offer go and, possibly with some satisfaction, countered with the suggestion that the two young men who had been working in the pathology laboratory on the surgical specimens he removed should be included in the authorship. As a result the three names Crohn, Ginzburg and Oppenheimer were associated, in alphabetical order. Had Berg been less preoccupied with other interests it would be known today as Berg's disease.

There are however other contenders for the honour of describing this new disease. 'I have pleasure in drawing attention to this condition which, I think, has not yet been fully described.' So said a Scottish surgeon from the Western Infirmary, Glasgow, with the awkward name of Dalziel – awkward because when spoken it loses most of its content and is pronounced 'deal'. The occasion was all but twenty years before Crohn's appearance at New Orleans; it was not dissimilar, for Dalziel was presenting his cases at the British equivalent of the American Medical Association meeting. The British Medical Association was meeting in Dalziel's home town, Glasgow, in July 1913. 'As far as I know the disease has not been previously described,' said the prudent Scot.

There was no hint of such caution in Crohn's account, nor was there a word of acknowledgement of earlier descriptions in the medical literature. The thought that there might be others who had seen ileitis does not appear to have crossed the minds of the Americans, unlike Dalziel who with his 'I think', and 'As far as I know' was clearly guarding against such possibility and protecting himself against the charge of plagiarism. This may seem odd, for Crohn himself was a thorough and knowledgeable investigator well versed in the relevant literature; to those who knew him and his ambition it might even seem suspect, but this would be an unfair and unworthy imputation.

Dalziel described a disease he called chronic intersitial enteritis; he had noticed that it affected various parts of the intestine, that it was not just confined to the terminal ileum. He saw it first in a patient who happened to be a doctor; that was in 1901. In all, he had operated upon nine patients by the time he presented his report; Berg, the reticent surgeon of Mount Sinai Hospital had operated upon thirteen of the fourteen upon whom the New York group based their paper in 1932.

In the face of these facts, why is it not Dalziel's disease? Probably because any interest aroused by Dalziel was almost certainly lost in the war years which followed when medical attention was rivetted on more pressing matters. His description would not have lingered in surgical minds to be recalled when the condition was encountered, as it must have been from time to time by the young surgeons who returned to civilian practice after the war. Dalziel died in 1924, aged 63. Why did he not pursue his observations further in the post-war years? Perhaps he felt he had done enough. The ambition to make his name as a surgeon was probably assuaged by a knighthood in 1917; he may have regarded that as sufficient recognition. Moreover the British Society of Gastroenterology had not yet been formed; that was to come in 1937, under the stimulus of a physician at Guy's Hospital, Dr Arthur Hurst, and a number of his contemporaries. Such a forum would have provided the opportunity, indeed the stimulus to present and discuss clinical problems of such uncertainty affecting the gut.

When it was rediscovered by Crohn it is clear from the discussion which followed his paper that the condition had been observed elsewhere in the United States. But on this side of the Atlantic when Crohn's paper was published and studied here, the condition was regarded as *recherché*, rare and of limited interest, of so little significance as to be printed in small type in the textbooks read by the medical students of those times. Had Crohn read the *British Medical Journal* of 1913 in which Dalziel's paper was published, and had he referred to it, there would no doubt have been a chance that regional enteritis, or chronic interstitial enteritis would have become known by the Scotsman's name. But there was nothing to direct him towards it; even Dalziel's fellow countrymen seemed to have fogotten its existence by 1932. Thus the seminal paper, the one which alerted doctors, appeared under the names of Crohn, Ginzburg and Oppenheimer in the *Journal of the American Medical Association* after the New Orleans début. From then on the medical profession was aware of this non-specific inflammatory disease and was on the look-out for the 'new', though rare, condition. Ironically two surgeons, Dalziel and Berg, had missed out on what was seen as essentially a surgical disease when it was first described, and the prize of immortal fame passed to a physician, with whom doubtless it will remain.

*

Crohn's disease is a 'non-specific' inflammatory disease; here is a piece of medical jargon which calls for explanation. It is an illness often associated with diarrhoea, though not always; in fact in only 60 per cent of patients does Crohn's ileitis present in this way. There are many other causes of

15

diarrhoea, and other diseases in which that symptom predominates; most are 'specific' because they have a recognisable cause. Dysentery is a *specific* inflammatory disease because it is caused by known bacterial organisms such as the *salmonella* (which cause typhoid) and *shigella*, sometimes by a parasite *entamoeba histolytica* (hence amoebic dysentery); and the tissues respond to bacterial or parasitic invasion by becoming inflamed. In fact inflammation is the response to any form of tissue damage and is therefore supposedly protective, though this scenario is blurred when an inflammatory response becomes chronic, that is long-standing, when the breakdown products of the tissue which result (tissue antigens) can cause an antibody response both prolonged and harmful. This mechanism may be part of what we observe in Crohn's disease causing its persistence, and fluctuating between periods of remission and recurrence.

Specific conditions such as those I have just mentioned by contrast tend to run a limited course; the patient might die but is far more likely to survive and the disease will disappear once the known cause has been overcome. That being said a distinction has to be made between acute and chronic specific disease. The bacilliary dysenteries are mostly acute and if not fatal will subside even without the appropriate specific treatment – usually an antibiotic, though not always. In cholera, for example, it is only necessary to ride out the storm by restoring into the veins the considerable fluid lost through diarrhoea; meanwhile, the body will deal with the bacteria.

It is true that any dysentery may become chronic if its cause remains and the condition therefore persists undetected. In another sense 'chronic' simply implies non-acute – we are not very exact in our semantics. Amoebic dysentery, for example, can present as a chronic disease for both these reasons.

Look at it in another way. There is much chronic diarrhoea in, say, Asia; mostly the causes are specific, being brought about by known bacteria, parasites or even viruses. The condition causing the illness does not fall into the category

16

of non-specific just because the cause, which is in fact lurking there to be detected, has not been demonstrated through lack of diagnostic facilities. Moreover more causes are known today than even a few years ago; whether or not this is simply a matter of our greater ability to detect micro-organisms through improvement in medical science, I do not know, though I suspect that some are new pathogens (causing abnormality in humans) and that there is an ever shifting scene in this respect. Bacteria, and viruses in particular, are readily capable of mutation. Today a bacterium, *campylobacter jejuni*, unheard of, indeed undiscovered, nine or so years ago, is now the commonest cause of hospital admission for diarrhoea in the UK and even in Bangladesh where so much else of greater antiquity is rife. While a small very mobile parasite, *lamblia giardia*, which infests the upper small intestine causing diarrhoea and which only a few years ago used to be an interesting variety, is now found as an almost universal contaminant of water supplies in the USSR. *Yersinia enterocolitica* is a recently recognised cause of terminal ileitis which simulates Crohn's disease so closely as to be an embarrassment at times; *yersinia*, a bacterium common in Scandinavia, is beginning to fan out into the Low Countries and is observed from time to time here.

There is, then, an ever shifting population of micro-organisms, some of which cause specific inflammatory bowel disease. A condition is said to be non-specific when the cause is undetermined; and there's the rub – as yet Crohn's disease has no identifiable cause.

There is another non-specific inflammatory bowel disease of older lineage – ulcerative colitis. Over a century ago two pathologists, Wilks and Moxon, gave the name to the disease. Of the many specimens of intestine which it was their misfortune to study there were some with appearances which did not present the known abnormal patterns associated with the dysenteries I have referred to. The nineteenth century was the great era of descriptive pathology, otherwise known as morbid anatomy, by which is simply meant: what looks different in an abnormal organ

17

or tissue. Medical science tends to advance on the most simple lines; the advent of anaesthetics in the middle of the century encouraged surgery so that operation specimens began to provide a boost to the pathologist. Living tissue immediately 'fixed' in formaldehyde after removal from a body gives a clearer microscopic picture than material removed at post-mortem when decomposition, initiated by self-destructive enzymes in the tissues, has been in progress for some time causing autolysis followed by bacterial breakdown. This particularly pertains in the large gut where in life bacteria abound but are restrained from attacking the bowel lining by special defence mechanisms there, mechanisms which fail on death. Even today when cadavers can be refrigerated to await post-mortem examination, autolytic changes do proceed in the gut to a degree which destroys the appearances observed in life. In the last century the study of pathology was hampered by a lack of total body refrigeration; surgical specimens therefore provided a stimulus to that science, particularly in the field of alimentary disease.

There was another reason why this non-specific condition had remained unidentified until then – a simple one. As in much of the third world today, in England then and Europe generally, diarrhoea due to one cause or another was rife. Those causes were infective, being easily passed from one individual to another in frequent epidemics, for hygiene as we know it was non-existent until piped water was supplied, and sewage contained and properly disposed of – a trend which started in the large towns in the nineteenth century and still has to be completed in some rural areas in the UK today. When infective diarrhoea was common, non-specific diarrhoea was obscured; so ulcerative colitis only became apparent as the tide of enteric infection receded, an experience which is being repeated in this century elsewhere. Not more than thirty years ago it was said that ulcerative colitis was unknown in the southern states of America such as Louisiana and in more recent times in Asia; but we now know that ulcerative colitis occurs in both regions.

18

Meanwhile, ironically, there is a resurgence of diarrhoea of specific infective origin both here and generally within the 'western' world, for though the drains still work, hygienic attitudes are changing socially, sexually and due to immigration. Another important reason lies in the methods employed in the mass production of meat now necessary to keep pace with the needs of increasing populations. Battery methods and crowded markets make for greater difficulty in controlling animal infections by organisms which may infest man. *Campylobacter* (more of which anon) infects us through imperfectly cooked poultry; it is particularly inclined to occur when chickens are deep-frozen and imperfectly defrosted before cooking, and is one example of this trend. A greater threat is posed in animal husbandry by using antibiotics in the feed in order to improve growth and weight, for this practice persists despite proscription. This pernicious habit encourages the growth in the gut of bacteria harmful to man, since the organisms develop resistance to the effects of the antibiotic; those organisms can all too easily contaminate a carcass and cause illness when ingested.

It is a pertinent fact that many a case of acute ulcerative colitis comes to our notice through admission to wards or hospitals set aside for communicable diseases – a title given to the full range of recognisable infections from specific fevers of childhood to the dysenteries – for many of the organisms mentioned induce inflammation in the large bowel, colitis in effect. The presentation and symptoms are the same in colitis whatever its cause, the predominant one being diarrhoea, a symptom inseparable from colonic inflammation. Although the intensity of diarrhoea may vary, it occurs to a greater or lesser degree whenever colitis is active.

That is one way in which ulcerative colitis differs from the other non-specific diseases; diarrhoea is not a *sine qua non* of Crohn's disease, one reason being that while ulcerative colitis always affects the large bowel, Crohn's disease does not. Indeed ulcerative colitis confines itself to the large intestine where it may extend throughout its length or settle in one area; Crohn's disease shows no such limitation, though it does have a predilection for the ileum. The areas involved in inflammation are seldom extensive, from which you may rightly surmise that Crohn's disease can be active at several different sites at one and the same time. By contrast, the lesions of ulcerative colitis are present in continuity along the gut.

*

The time has come when we should look at intestinal function, which has some part to play in the presentation of any disease of the alimentary system. Mouth, gullet and stomach matter less in this respect since they are only rarely involved in Crohn's disease and never in ulcerative colitis. Even when Crohn's disease develops at any of those sites it has little effect upon mastication or swallowing, it does not impede the passage of food down the gullet or impair the churning mill provided by the stomach, where acid is secreted and mixed in with gastric contents to provide a uniform pabulum to be squirted out into the gut beyond, the site of the greatest activity of digestion and absorption.

Into the very first part of the intestinal tube, the duodenum, a juice flows partly from the liver in the form of bile and partly from the pancreas. This juice is alkaline and so neutralises the acidity imparted by the stomach enabling protein digestion to get under way with the aid of pancreatic secretion (which is activated by acidity). Proteins, with fats and carbohydrates, are broken down further into their component molecules by numerous enzymes formed in cells in the jejunal wall designed solely for this purpose, the jejunum being the next section along from the duodenum. The activity is considerable and the achievement remarkable, for apart from the volume of fluid which enters the duodenum from the stomach each day, that is about seven to eight litres (approximately 15 pints), there is a considerable flux of water in and out of the tissue lining the intestine, part and parcel of the intricate chemistry of absorption. Sodium particles (ions) are pushed in and out of the lining (mucosa) by a sort of rocking or rotating pump mechanism in the outer envelope of the cell, the pump

20

being activated by energy it receives from sugar molecules. So water pours out into the space in the centre, the lumen as we call it, and is carried back in again, taking with it ions of potassium, while more complex molecules are pushed and nudged along into mucosal cells from one side and out through less than microscopic holes (electronmicroscopic in fact) on the other, and so on into the blood stream.

The actual quantity of water involved in this two way flux is great; therein lies the secret of cholera. The *vibrio*, which is the family name of the bacterium responsible for cholera, secretes a special antienzyme which switches off the powerful physiochemical mechanism designed to enable the water to be returned from the jejunal cavity back into the blood stream. In fact it acts by a very subtle piece of biochemical skullduggery, for the antienzyme it produces mimics the enzyme which the mucosal cell itself produces to switch off that rocking pump for its own purpose; the cholera toxin may even be identical with it. So the cholera vibrio gets in and takes over to its advantage and to man's disadvantage, often gravely so, through an act of internal sabotage. Like a bore in an estuary, a flood of water too great to be absorbed or contained below, rushes down the alimentary canal and so out as rather impure water containing the sodium and potassium which should have been absorbed with it. Meanwhile the patient dries up and begins to droop like a neglected plant – becomes, in a word, dehydrated. Until the physiochemistry of cholera became unravelled recently, it was a highly lethal illness; all that is now required to save the patient's life is to put back into his veins a large volume of saline and wait until the cholera vibrio is overcome, as it will be by natural mechanisms within that mucosa. Treatment was less effective when we relied upon attacking the vibrio itself with antibiotics. One rather academic question remains: what biological advantage does the great flux present to the vibrio? We do not know.

To return to a less turbulent state; with all systems working, what is left from the food as it passes to the ileum? First, where is the ileum? If you were to look at the small intestine – indeed you may have done so in poultry or an animal such as rabbit when preparing either for the pot – you would not be able to lay your finger on any one spot and say above here is jejunum, below is ileum. The character of the small intestine changes gradually from beginning to end as the function required of it changes; less is demanded of the end, the ileal end, than the beginning because so much has already been achieved by the jejunum. The bile plays a special role with the salts it contains in reducing surface tension and thus enabling globules of fat to become smaller and emulsified to enable digestion; it is retained until the ileum is reached, where most of it is absorbed and circulated back to the liver. Also in the lower reaches vitamin B_{12}, important to the formation of red blood cells, is absorbed; loss of function of the terminal ileum can lead to anaemia of a particular form – clearly a matter of importance in Crohn's disease though not in ulcerative colitis. Water absorption continues throughout the gut so that that also is part of ileal function though to a far lesser degree than in the jejunum; one and a half litres (about 3 pints) in volume passes on out of the small intestine each day through the ileo-caecal junction into the colon.

What about that 'mucosa' I have mentioned? It is the inner lining of any part of the alimentary system from the mouth to within three quarters of an inch of the ultimate orifice at the anus. In principle the function of mucosa anywhere is to enable absorption of what is required by the body while at the same time giving protection from any noxious thing presented to it. Clearly where absorption is greatest that protection must be safest since the risk of something unwanted slipping in is more likely there. Let us look at this in different areas.

No actual absorption occurs in the mouth or gullet but the mucosal lining of those organs nevertheless have to contribute to that activity by facilitating absorption further on; so lubricant is provided in the only form the body knows – mucus, which is poured out in abundance from salivary glands in the mouth to be well mixed in by mastication, and carried down the gullet where additional mucus is provided by similar small glands. Because of this limited function, the lining membrane is relatively thin compared with what is to follow.

Not so in the stomach, where the mucosa is at its thickest – as anyone who enjoys tripe must be aware; for much fluid, acid and pepsin has to be added to the mix by the stomach. If like a surgeon you were able to hold the jejunum between your fingers and compare it with the ileum you would observe that the jejunum is noticeably thicker – due to the greater digestive activity there necessitating more active mucosa. There is also the other protective function represented in that mucosa by myriads of cells lying apparently haphazardly, unconnected in any recognisable architectural pattern which is an obvious feature of the glandular arrangement of the digestive cells. These loose cells, which constitute what is known as the stroma, seem to vary in density and number. They are those very cells which are to be seen agglomerating at a site of infection and inflammation; indeed they are inflammatory cells.

Thus at all times the mucosa appears to be mildly inflamed; if you were to look at the tissue underlying the flat surface cells of the skin you would see no suspicion of inflammation, or if you did you would know something was wrong. But under the column-like epithelial cells which form the surface of gut mucosa it is very different, so that it can be difficult to draw the line between what is right and proper and what constitutes active inflammation. The explanation is simple: inflammatory cells have to be present, constantly on guard along the gut, because there is incessant invasion from its lumen of antigens, those noxious molecules in the form of bacteria or of sensitising protein. There are little spaces between the epithelial cells to allow what is needed to pass through; the foreigners can get in as well. Nothing can stop them; but inside the epithelial breakwater, inflammatory cells have been placed to pounce upon bacteria or form immune reactions to cope with toxins and other foreign proteins. A heavy invasion requires a bigger response and this is to be seen under the microscope as a stroma more densely packed with cells.

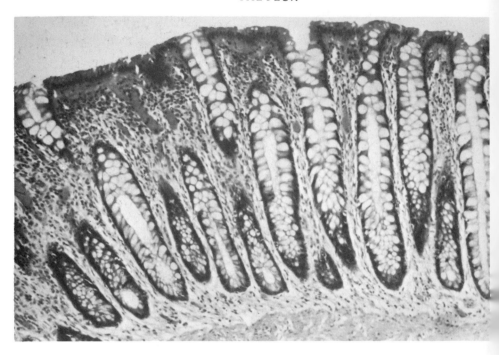

Figure 1. Here is a photograph of normal bowel lining – the mucosa – seen through the microscope. The clear space at the top is the inside – the lumen – of the gut. The faint strip at the bottom is the muscle at the base of the mucosa. In between lies the mucosa, along the upper edge of which is a strip of epithelial cells lying cheek by jowl, their nuclei standing out darkly. The glands – the crypts – are the most obvious feature, dipping into the supporting tissue – the stroma – their walls formed by the same epithelial cells but now displaying large blobs of mucus which they are manufacturing, to be passed into the cavity of the gland and so to the lumen of the gut above. The stroma forming the background is a *mélange* of round cells committed to immuno-logical defence.

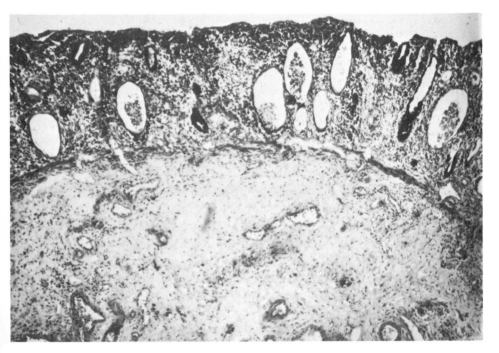

Figure 2. This shows what happens when the mucosa becomes inflamed (the magnification is approximately half that seen in figure 1). The normal architecture is lost. A number of glands have become little abscesses, ballooned by distension with pus, while many glands have disappeared altogether. There is a noticable increase of the cells in the surrounding stroma. As colitis progresses the thickness of the mucosa becomes diminished by ulceration even to the point of being lost altogether in the severe case.

Down in the colon the mucosa becomes thin for it has less to do – absorb water and salts, and get rid of excess potassium; that is just about all except, of course, to produce some more lubricant, for as the colonic contents pass from the right to the left side and so out, so in these final stages of water absorption they become less fluid, then actually formed and solid. Food was taken in solid and needed lubrication; faeces are also solid and need lubrication to help move them out – one reason why mucus can be a feature of constipation; more lubricant is required. As for those immune complexes, they are needed all the more in the colon, which teems with bacteria in its lumen.

It is odd that bacteria are not present in normal small intestine anywhere from the stomach onwards – at least not in sufficient quantity to be demonstrable by ordinary bacteriological means. That is a tribute to the defense mechanisms, which get away to a flying start in the stomach because the acidity there is anathema to many organisms. Suddenly it seems as though these devices lose their grip in the large bowel. But it is all a matter of economy of effort; there is no longer any need to pour protective inflammatory cells into the lumen to sweep the area clean of contamination, so why bother? Bacteria in the small gut would compete for the foodstuff being digested there; by the time the colon is reached man has taken all he needs leaving only some water and salt to be gathered, and bacteria are hardly going to quibble with him for possession of that.

The point that intestinal bacteria would enjoy the sugars, fats and amino-acids to be found in the small intestine is sometimes brought home all too forcibly to those who like to eat the jerusalem artichoke. This vegetable presents carbohydrate in a form unusual to man – inulin. Ingestion of artichokes is soon followed by an embarrassing excess of intestinal gas, probably because most of us are not well endowed with inulinase, the enzyme necessary for its digestion, if at all. Some of the sugar then passes on to the ever avaricious hordes lurking in the large gut, to be utilised by them with, as a by-product, intestinal gas in excess.

There is evidence also from gut abnormality of the untoward effect of bacteria when they gain access to the small intestine; normally they are restrained by a flap valve which prevents reflux of intestinal content at the ileocaecal junction. A short circuit operation between small and large intestine will overcome the efficacy of this barrier, as does retardation of the intestinal flow by partial obstruction – both important factors in the Crohn's story. Under these circumstances bacteria colonise the small intestine to cause malnutrition because of competition from the bacteria and the impairment of absorption they bring about.

Gut bacteria are harmless in the right place – the large intestine. Indeed they are a positive advantage there, where they pursue the cycle of life, albeit a mini-cycle. Just as bacterial decomposition is essential in terrestial ecology, so they are needed in our gut to decompose epithelial cells, the enterocytes. These very active cells form the protective outer layer of the mucosa, separating it from the gut canal; that layer covers a considerable acreage for it is deeply enfolded. Enterocytes are multitudinous, are very active and wear out quickly. The worn out shells are constantly shed into the gut to be swept onwards with the food they have helped to digest, to be digested in their turn by the bacteria in the colon. You could imagine that the works might become clogged up otherwise.

It would be wrong to suppose from what has been said that gut contents pour down the alimentary canal like a stream under its own volition. From beginning to end the food is propelled along by contractions of the gut, sometimes in fits and starts where intermittency is appropriate to the function of the area. Food in the stomach has to be mixed, so it is moved backwards and forwards within that organ with churning effect; a little of the contents is ejected from time to time through the valve separating stomach from duodenum, the pyloric sphincter. From then on progress is continuous until the large intestine is reached; there, in order to extract as much fluid as possible from what has become a faecal stream, an intermittency of contraction is again imparted to provide a to and fro movement so that as much of the contents come into contact with the water-absorbing mucosal surface as possible. The bowels open when everything contained in the last part of the colon and the rectum is shot out in one continuous action.

All this activity is achieved by muscle surrounding the mucosa in two layers, the outer lying lengthways and the inner at right angles to this in circular fashion, the two being co-ordinated by nerves which are part of a nervous system that neither lets you know what is going on nor allows you to dictate the action it should ordain: the autonomic nervous system. As with the mucosa, the muscle is more prominent where contractions have to be stronger, yet another reason why the wall of the stomach is thicker than that in the intestine. But the changes brought about by inflammatory bowel disease can interfere with all this, as we shall see.

2 The gut disturbed

What is diarrhoea? The significance of this symptom may seem obvious; however, the interpretation of the word varies considerably. To most people it seems to imply that the bowels are being opened more often than usual. And there is a snag, for what is the normal frequency of stool? We have been brought up to think that it is correct to open our bowels once daily, in the morning. No doubt this may be the normal state for most of us, but such is individual variation that it is not uncommon for perfectly healthy individuals to have their bowels open every other day, conversely some do so twice a day. Wider variations from the common experience of a daily bowel motion are not so common; though an evacuation of stool every third day is the lifetime experience of a few and there are more who will evacute normally after each main meal in the day. There is therefore no absolute figure of normality to provide a common experience; diarrhoea represents an increase in daily bowel actions over what happens to be usual for that individual. That is not the end of the matter; many interpret as diarrhoea the passage of a soft or fluid stool without any associated increase in frequency. In fact most people with diarrhoea usually suffer from both an increase in the number of evacuations and looseness of the stool.

Colitis spells diarrhoea, but not in the manner described in the last chapter. The origin of the watery stools of cholera, traditionally described as 'rice-water stools' – the opacity being caused by mucus together with cells shed from the mucosa – the source of these cataracts is located far away from the orifice through which they emerge. For cholera is an example of small bowel diarrhoea. The mechanisms of absorption need only to be disturbed, and this can be caused in a number of ways not necesssarily through the fault of an external agency such as the cholera vibrio.

Purgation by the use of simple chemicals such as magnesium sulphate, is an obvious example in point. The sulphate part of Epsom salts receives scant attention from the avid mucosal cell seeking out the simple chemicals needed by the body. Both components of common or garden salt, sodium and chloride, are basic to our biochemical processes; so both are absorbed. Magnesium is as essential as sodium, though required in far smaller quantity, but the sulphate part is not. If this sulphate radical could be broken down to the elements of which it is composed, oxygen and sulphur, the oxygen ions would no doubt be made use of, but the sulphur would not, for sulphur has no place in the body's economy in terms of electrolyte activity – the activity, that is, which creates the electrical charges indispensible to cell activity, the power which makes them (and us) go.

Sulphur is vital for us but not in this form – only when assimilated in one of that multitude of amino-acids which, combined together, make up a molecule of protein. Incorporated within an amino-acid known as cystein, sulphur can be absorbed into the body, but in a way in which it loses its identity and so can do no harm. Quite the reverse in fact

29

because it gives an identity to cystein and a special purpose, that amino-acid being an essential part of the protein structure of the outer waterproof layer of the skin and of hair.

So the body takes its supply of sulphur ready packaged in the form in which it is needed, and sulphur on its own serves no general purpose. Why bother to waste time on a special mechanism to enable it to pass through the mucosal cell lining in the way that sodium is pushed through? That would be an expensive frill in terms of the economy of cellular activity. So the sulphate part of magnesium sulphate is ignored as it passes along on its way through the bowel. But this is done at some cost. The sulphate continues to embrace its partner magnesium (or it may transfer to any sodium particles which are knocking around) in order to combine in a molecule which can be handled in solution. Magnesium (or sodium) sulphate holds on to water in the gut contents so that its concentration, together with the other salts dissolved thus, remains in equilibrium with the concentration of salts within the cells and the tissue spaces of the body. As a result water is held back within the gut, increasing the volume of its contents, and overwhelming the capacity of the colon to absorb it, so that the stool becomes fluid. The more Epsom salts taken the more fluid is excreted through the bowel.

This purgative process also plays a part in that form of diarrhoea endured by patients with coeliac disease and the related condition of sprue. Clinically these conditions are linked by a common feature: the diarrhoea is fatty – the result of defective mucosal cells in the jejunum. The defect is brought about either by a congenital or acquired sensitivity to gluten and this affects those sensitive cells. Gluten is a conglomerate mass, rather than an identifiable chemical, left behind when starch has been extracted from wheat; it is gluten which gives dough its consistency. This defect can also be caused by parasites harbouring in the small intestine. In the happy pink days of our far flung empire, 'colonials' out east were sometimes less happily afflicted by tropical sprue, the causes of which are still not entirely clear but which was often associated with parasitic infestation –

intestinal worms and the like. The colonials have left but not the parasites; steatorrhoea – fatty diarrhoea – still troubles the indigenous people of tropical parts. How does this come about?

In normal circumstances the jejunal mucosa seen through a scanning electron microscope is a beautiful sight – like a sea anemone; fronds wave and undulate gently with the flow of the fluid which bathes them. Between the villi, as the fronds are called, are pits leading to caverns, or crypts. The epithelial cells which provide the surface of the mucosa do not stay in the same place; they are formed at the bottom of the crypts and are constantly on the move, flowing in sheets towards the tip of the villus where old age overcomes them and they drop off to be swept away into the gut and devoured by bacteria below. The cells present in miniature what happens to the total organism in life; just as disease may shorten life so will disorder reduce the active span of these cells. Cells weakened by gluten sensitivity for example die before their time so that the villi shorten and become stunted, the acreage of digestive surface is reduced, with associated loss of digestive function; malabsorption follows.

The first item to be affected is fat normally broken down to fatty acids and emulsified, the rather bulky globules then being passed into the mucosal cell and out the other side, to be carried away and distributed through the body in pipes specially designed for the purpose. When fat is undigested or only partially so, the intestinal stream moves it on, so that the unaltered fat is all too soon to be found where it can no longer be assimilated, for the length of gut capable of fat absorption is limited. To make matters worse, bacteria appear where they were never intended; for some obscure reason the upper reaches of the small bowel become colonised by bacteria, possibly because the protective function of the mucosa is disturbed by the general affliction. Indeed those inflammatory cells in the stroma between the epithelium and the muscle proliferate, but whether *post* or *propter hoc* it is difficult to say. Whichever the case, some of the bacteria that arrive are chasing the unaltered fat,

31

turning it to their advantage and to the disadvantage of their host, since they create abnormal fatty acids which cannot be absorbed. So the original defect is compounded and steatorrhoea follows, though this does not fully account for the diarrhoea the patient suffers. The changes in the mucosal architecture, including oedematous swelling, probably deform the cells in such a manner as to distort the spaces between them. As a result the normal flow of sodium and water in and out of the body through the surface of the mucosa is hindered, thus adding to the volume of the alimentary stream, compromising the situation and enhancing the diarrhoeic effect.

Jejunal cells are sensitive to noxious agents in addition to those of sprue and coeliac disease. Of the many wounds we inflict upon ourselves with alcohol jejunal damage may be the least obvious. Nonetheless it occurs in a brief, acute form recognisable in the abdominal symptoms of a hangover; in that period the stool may be loose, pale in colour due to the presence of unaltered fat, and flushing imperfectly down the pan. This embarrassing difficulty reflects the ability of fat to float on water.

There are, too, osmotic diarrhoeas due to biochemical deficiencies of the *milieu interieur* which may be as explosive as anything Epsom salts can achieve, disturbance of carbohydrate digestion being a case in point. Sugars are highly soluble and so exert an osmotic effect, which is one reason why so much water pours out of the stomach wall to greet a meal: the substances in solution have to be brought into osmotic balance with fluid in the tissues which surround them. Removal of the stomach in part or in whole, a surgical operation less frequently performed now than it was twenty five years ago, proves how important this is, for all those substances like salts and sugars which are brought into solution in the stomach or diluted there in order to equalise the osmotic pressure with that inside the body, are shot too quickly into the small intestine before this equalisation can be fully achieved. Dilution has to continue in the jejunum which thus becomes dilated by the increasing volume with untoward effects – abdominal discomfort, distension and fainting. The whole sequence has been disturbed so that the bulk moves rapidly on, often presenting the colon with more fluid than it can cope with. In addition sugars appear in the large bowel where they cannot be absorbed; they continue to hold water there until all is passed as a fluid stool. So the 'dumping' which may follow removal of the stomach can also cause watery diarrhoea after every meal.

Not dissimilar is the way in which diarrhoea comes about in those who cannot digest all the sugar in milk. As its name implies lactose is that sugar; it is formed by the conjunction of molecules of two sugars, glucose and galactose. Unlike glucose, lactose cannot be absorbed, which creates no problem for most of us since our ever provident mucosal cells make the appropriate enzyme, lactase, to split the sugar into its absorbable component parts. But for some it is different; they are born with an inability to manufacture lactase. For them lactose is no less of a cathartic than Epsom salts. The water which has to dilute the lactose in order to retain osmotic balance is carried to the large bowel where bacteria break down the lactose, but too late since sugars cannot be absorbed there, and the two molecules of sugar make a greater demand for water than the simple parent molecule would have done, thus increasing the osmotic load and making matters worse. Fortunately the cure is simple – avoid milk and milk products; that the condition is rare may be fortunate in one respect but less so in another since it tends, therefore, not to be borne in mind and may be overlooked as a cause of repeated and unexplained diarrhoea.

*

In the days of my youth we used to suffer from attacks of what was called food-poisoning; the phrase is often used today. The term used to puzzle me since with youthful literalism I tended to regard a poison as some noxious chemical. The fact that the vomiting and diarrhoea were heralded by fever should have given me the clue that food-poisoning was probably an infection. But how could a boy be expected to know, particularly in those distant days when relatively few of the microbial causes we recognise today were known? We know little enough at the present time, but we are aware that bacteria are not the only culprits. Viruses have now been incriminated; specific types have been extracted from stools and identified by electronmicroscopy. Unlike the viruses which cause 'flu their cousins marauding in the gut are difficult to maintain in captivity: they will not grow in the laboratory. It is easy to grow bacteria; they can be provided with small dishes of agar – a jelly extracted from seaweed – laced with the appropriate nutrients and tucked up in a little incubator to keep warm. Sometimes oxygen has to be excluded, in particular for the organisms which usually inhabit the colon; since most of these are anaerobic, they cannot survive in an atmosphere containing oxygen.

A virus is virtually nothing but nuclear material and seems to be limited in its capabilities; for example it cannot make use of the agar ground in the way a bacterium can to provide for its needs. In a sense a bacterium is more like a plant and a virus like an animal, a shark in particular, for a virus feeds avidly on meat – tissue cells, that is, which can be cultured in sheets and, thus formed, used in their turn to farm the virus. We can tell when bacteria are growing on agar plates for they develop into colonies which can be seen with the naked eye. Viruses do not congregate happily in this way, and they remain invisible; the only evidence that they are living in the cell culture is the disappearance of those cells which can otherwise be observed readily with light magnification and which reveal the presence of viruses by turning up their toes and dying. Special preparations can then be made in order to demonstrate the presence of the virus with the aid of electron microscopy.

The respiratory viruses can be grown in this way so that quite a lot has been learnt about them; but we have been unsuccessful in cultivating the few we have been able to identify from patients inflicted with vomiting and diarrhoea; we have not yet found the tempting morsel for enteric viruses. Mostly, these viruses seem to attack children or babies; the family of rotavirus was only demonstrated in 1973, but it is now known to be common around the world particularly in children's wards and nurseries. Adults are less affected both by the infection and its severity, possibly because many have been infected in childhood and so have acquired immunity. There are others like the rotavirus; it would be tedious and pointless to reel off their names, more particularly because we suspect there are numerous species of viruses as yet unidentified which could be responsible for the gastroenteritis we all suffer in the not infrequent epidemics developing in winter. This suspicion is based upon the fact that bacteria which might be responsible are often conspicuous by their absence on these occasions. One other point is worth noting. The attentions of the rotavirus are not confined to man; it infects other animal species, in particular their young, as in the human disease; in fact, rotavirus was first detected in calves. Where calves in herds are infected it is possible to demonstrate the virus in the cows, which raises disturbing thoughts as regards the source of epidemics, but at the same time indicates a possible animal species in which a vaccine against rotavirus might be raised.

It would probably be incorrect to regard viral gastroenteritis as food poisoning, since it seems that the infection on many occasions has not come via the food. No doubt enterotoxic viruses can enter that way, for anything is possible; but the way epidemics develop appears to indicate aerial spread, by droplet infection – a term sufficiently descriptive to require no further elaboration. But here again uncertainty prevails, greatly to our disadvantage since we do not know which way to turn to avoid the invisible blow.

A little more is known about how a virus causes diarrhoea. Although the intestine has been almost a closed book to those who need to discover its secrets, its shape and appearance can be displayed by x-rays; but that only gives information in the gross. One way to improve on this is by taking a sample of the lining of the jejunum for study; the trick is achieved by getting the patient to swallow a tube, of a bore just sufficient to contain controls to trigger off a little knife in a small capsule at the end, and then retrieving the

35

small piece of mucosa cut off. This biopsy can be studied under the microscope and even the electronmicroscope. From such observations during epidemics two deductions can be drawn. The jejunal mucosa is abnormal in the way that I have previously described; hand in hand with that, impairment of enzyme production from the mucosal cells has been demonstrated in the acute phase of viral diarrhoea. Ergo: the diarrhoea is due to brief impairment of sugar and fat absorption. This has been confirmed by examining the stools. Does this come about because the viral particles settle there, in the jejunum? Very probably; little holes appear in the mucosal cells where they may lurk, for viruses destroy cells by invading them and not by secreting a toxin.

The production of a toxin is the prerogative of bacteria, most of them being able to elaborate a poison (so the term food-poisoning has some cogency) and deliver it to the enterocytes – the epithelial cells of the mucosa. Clearly the bacteria have got to be within range; *escherichia coli*, a large group which provides many of the bacteria which live in the colon in happy coexistence with us without causing trouble, turn against us. By some means *E coli* contrive to work their way into the small intestine, the enterocytes being their target. If the toxin they exude is to be effective they have to remain close by in the face of the forceful peristaltic flow, its volume increased by extra fluid. So they develop a special ability to stick to the surface of the epithelial cells. In doing so they display one of the tricks by which bacteria can adapt to adverse circumstances and yet survive.

Bacteria come in all shapes and sizes, but they are fundamentally the same in that a single bacterium comprises one cell containing a nucleus of genetic material, the template for survival and reproduction, surrounded by cell sap, the cytoplasm, all being enveloped in an outer membrane. A bacterium is like any other cell with the exception that it lives independently. Although it can reproduce itself – and it has to – the enterocyte against which the bacterium pits itself cannot survive on its own. In its nucleus the bacterium is endowed with the wherewithal to get by; the nucleus instructs the cell components found in the cytoplasm what to do and keeps them ticking over.

But bacteria are very vulnerable to change in their environment, which may suddenly become hostile particularly with antibiotics around. So they need to adapt. Not all can do so; for example, the *streptococcus haemolyticus*, the cause of scarlet fever amongst other serious illnesses, was *the* scourge of my youth. Now it is hardly ever encountered; penicillin put paid to it. In the heyday of the streptococcus the staphylococcus was of less significance; it mostly caused pimples and at its worst boils and carbuncles. Today the staphylococcus has pride of place, although at first it succumbed to penicillin as the streptococcus did. Penicillin is now inactive against the staphylococcus because the bacterium has been able to adapt. It took on special gear in the form of additional nuclear material to be found lying around in colonies of staphylococci. These little parcels of hereditary material, known as plasmids, are worth their weight in gold – like grasping an ace to trump with. For with the plasmid on board the staphylococcus possesses the code to start making an enzyme to destroy penicillin. Being genetic material the additional code provided by plasmids is passed on to subsequent generations. Thus forms of staphylococci capable of resisting antibiotics are ensured while those without plasmid protection lose out and disappear for ever – or almost, for those with plasmids in their grasp may sometimes lose their grip and revert to the unprotected type.

And it is by the misuse of antibiotics, prescribing them unnecessarily, that we create resistant forms of bacteria – the most serious and blatant therapeutic abuse of our times.

To return to *E coli*: for the most part it is a harmless organism which does us a service in the colon devouring the detritus, the garbage of worn out cells. It can however widen its scope, if need be, by taking to itself a plasmid, or even two – one to enable it to adhere to the small intestinal wall and stay put, the other to provide the ability to manufacture toxin designed to cause the intestinal cells to yield fluid and nutrients without destroying them. Meanwhile the human host harbouring this struggle suffers diarrhoea.

Members of the coliform family take on many roles, from acute gastroenteritis in infants to traveller's diarrhoea. An attack of diarrhoea is a common experience for those who go abroad, particularly to the warm climates of Africa, Asia and the far East. There are numerous causes; it may be due to parasites such as *giardia lamblia* but as often as not the attack has been caused by recolonisation with a different breed of coliform bacteria. The form which predominates varies from place to place, from one continent to another, from Africa to the far East, from North America to Mexico; in a new environment we tend to rid ourselves of what we carried in our gut and take on the local brand; sometimes the change brings on diarrhoea. Which raises the question as to why the local inhabitants are not afflicted if the traveller is. The answer would seem to lie in immunity. Perhaps all coliforms are intrinsically harmful but the toxic activities of those we harbour are held in check by immunity of long standing; we just come to terms with those we take on board. In such immunity must lie the answer to the treatment of traveller's diarrhoea, which when due to coliform exchange should aim at easing the symptom of diarrhoea rather than snubbing the coliform with chemicals such as antibiotics. It is even better to prevent an attack through simple precautions – which will also help guard against more serious and prolonged dangers, such as dysentery or parasitic infestation – by abstaining from water from the cold tap (even for brushing the teeth), ice in drinks and raw and uncooked food, particularly salads or fruit which cannot be peeled. Wine and canned beer are fairly safe, but bottled beverages can be contaminated and have even been known to cause typhoid. The safest drink is a hot beverage, more particularly when the water has been boiled by yourself. You are most at danger from food you buy in the streets: cafés and restaurants are more risky than private homes. Even a swim in fresh water presents hazards. In addition these precautions will help the traveller to avoid the more serious possibility of hepatitis against which antibiotics offer no protection at all.

The objections to taking antimicrobial drugs in advance to avoid traveller's diarrhoea or dysentery are twofold and considerable. This is an indiscriminate use of antibiotics, an abuse, as already explained, which we must learn to eschew. And what antibiotic would one select? To make a choice can only be to draw a bow at a venture, for no single antibiotic is capable of dealing with every microbe. For a time a drug known as Entero-Vioform, an oxyquinoline, was popular for it was thought to have a general inhibitory effect on bacteria without the selectivity which is a feature of most antibiotics. But it proved to be no panacea. If it had been, its very success would have raised more serious problems; for what happens if the gut is sterilised? It must become recolonised and the organisms which begin to reappear may be those we least wish to entertain. Indeed there has been evidence that bacteria of the typhoid group, the salmonella, flourish more often in travellers who have received oxyquinolines than those who have not – a testimony to their partial yet dubious success.

Traveller's diarrhoea is the most likely cause of a tummy upset for anyone on the move, though any of the more specific dysenteries may be the cause. Half of those who travel to developing countries from the USA develop the trots, of insufficient severity to deter the prospective traveller but enough to cause a third of those afflicted inconvenience to the extent of having to alter plans or even retire to bed. Since the bacterium responsible is most commonly one of the *E coli* family any of which may be capable of producing a toxin to attack the gut it inhabits, it is understandable that antibiotics with an affinity for this organism, like doxycycline, are still being recommended for prophylactic use. Nevertheless, although there may be special reasons why an individual needs to be protected, preventive treatment with antimicrobial agents should not be used indiscriminately in the hope of protecting everyone who leaves his own shores. Not only does this practice discourage the normal bowel flora to the advantage of organisms better avoided, but the indiscriminate use of antibiotics simply for this purpose can endanger the body in other ways by creating resistance to drugs which might be needed for infections like typhus and malaria.

Mostly, the watery diarrhoea will subside in two to three days and other symptoms – fever, colic and vomiting – will abate. It is only rarely that the unpleasantness persists for longer and causes any serious degree of prostration. So the strategy is to weather the storm until it abates while relieving the symptoms as far as possible. There are a variety of drugs which meet this purpose from simple codeine phosphate to the opiates, or more modern developments like diphenoxylate (Lomotil) and loperamide (Imodium). These are not taken in anticipation but when the first signs of trouble start; it is my personal experience that diphenoxylate, for instance, will actually put paid to colic, diarrhoea and nausea if taken at the outset and maintained for twenty four to forty eight hours.

Who would be foolish enough to encourage the thief in the night or the violent intruder intent upon trespass against his person? Taking an antibiotic as a bow at a venture against a chance encounter with an unknown organism is little different. The practice can only tend to drive an offending bacterium into resistant form to do battle on another day with the aid of a plasmid or two, and so cause persistent symptoms. Failing that, while causing little disturbance to the erstwhile traveller the offending organism may turn his gut to its own account as a launching pad for further excursion into the community through the carrier-state; but more of that later.

---

3 Dangers lurking in food

The chance of picking up an infection which may affect the gut is becoming increasingly common. To take one group of bacteria as an example of the problem – *salmonella*; these are the organisms responsible for typhoid and paratyphoid, the enteric fevers. Bacteria more commonly responsible for food poisoning referred to in the last chapter begin to take effect within twenty four hours or less, occasionally rather longer. But the typhoid and paratyphoid organisms seem to need to incubate for ten days to two weeks before they get under way, when the illness often presents with fever, and though diarrhoea may shortly follow it is less acute than in food poisoning, in which vomiting and diarrhoea predominate.

But that is only half the story, less in fact. The typhoid group are those members of the sizeable salmonella family which choose to live with man; there are others which prefer to infest animals of their special choice from among sheep, pigs, cattle, hens and horses to name only a few; and there are a host of salmonellae which have not adapted to any one species – seventeen thousand different types floating about looking for a patron, as it were. Fortunate for us, you might think, to have attracted the specific attention of only a few; this is not so however, for the variety which prefer to inhabit animals and the unadapted members among the salmonellae are also capable of making us ill by way of food poisoning leading to diarrhoea and vomiting starting within twelve to twenty four hours, associated with malaise, headache, the gripes and fever. Very occasionally they go further and emulate their typhoid cousins by getting through and beyond the bowel lining into the blood to produce a generalised infection.

Above all salmonellae inhabit the gut, their natural home in the vertebrate kingdom they infest; moreover, they can do so in a 'carrier state'. In other words they can get taken on board and live like all those other organisms in the large bowel causing no trouble to their host, but unlike them a potential danger to others. Faecal contamination from a carrier can start an epidemic, as happened in a big way in the late 1930s when a man unknown to be a carrier was employed in the renovation of a well at Addington which fed the Croydon water supply. An epidemic of typhoid suddenly exploded afflicting four hundred or more of the inhabitants of that town causing death in no less than twenty per cent. Although typhoid is fortunately rare in countries with sewage disposal, here was a case where drinking water had been contaminated by excrement from one man. Much, if not most of the world's population must still be at considerable risk not just from the water they drink but from any food eaten raw, such as lettuce, which should be washed free of contamination during preparation.

There are the animal carriers: that pet terrapin may be harbouring a salmonella to contaminate the fingers of whoever cleans out its tank, or worse, the crocks in the kitchen sink if that is the most convenient place to empty the tank. This may appear far-fetched, but it does represent one of the many ways in which salmonella can crop up unexpectedly. More important is the possible infestation of animals which provide our food, in particular pigs and poultry. Human contamination is less likely to occur from animals which are actually infected, since the trouble should be obvious at the slaughter house, than from the animal carriers which are not detected.

Trouble lies in the fact that the circumstances of modern living in no way ameliorate or offset the enormous potential for harm salmonella present; quite the reverse. In the days of my youth, fifty or so years ago, the problems presented by an outbreak of food poisoning were relatively easy to solve. In order to bring an outbreak under control there is detective work to be done. We first have to find out which food was contaminated, then trace the supply of the incriminated item to its source where it should be possible to indentify the presence of the bacteria which were responsible, and how they got into the food. Food distribution in those days was a local affair, confined to the local farmer or small-holder and the butcher who distributed it to his customers residing within the locality. Admittedly food regulations of those days were less stringent than now so that the community was more reliant upon the sense of responsibility of these individuals or, conversely, subject to their slovenliness. But consider the changes brought about by modern marketing and international trading. Take the example of the sudden appearance of a salmonella previously unheard of on the international scene.

In 1969 *salmonella agona* began to be isolated from the diarrhoeic stools of patients with food poisoning; this particular member of the family had hitherto rarely been found in humans. That fact was odd enough in itself to raise the suspicion that an individual item of food was being contaminated. But odder still was the grand geographical scale on which *agona* was making its debut – in the USA and UK, both places where isolated human infection had been reported occasionally before, and also in the Netherlands and Israel where it had never been discovered previously. By 1972 this former *inconnu* had become the eighth most common organism responsible for food poisoning in the USA, infecting 500 patients there in that year, while in the UK it had risen to second place with 700 cases. The mystery of its source remained: then, in the same year, some American public health doctors had a stroke of luck.

An outbreak occurred in Paragould, a small town in Arkansas of just over 10,000 souls; this was traced to one restaurant where the poultry supply was incriminated. The chase was then on. It led to a large poultry supplier in Mississippi and to what the birds had to eat. By 1972 the world demand for fish meal to be used for animal feed had increased to such an extent that the USA along with other maritime countries had had to look beyond their own coastal waters to supplement their stocks. Peru was making up that deficit and, indeed, supplying forty to sixty per cent of the world's needs. There, in the fish meal, the doctors found their quarry transported from Peruvian waters.

Like most bacteria, salmonella is killed by heat; proper defrosting and thorough cooking will destroy the organism. The restaurant in Paragould did their job properly, there was no question of imperfect cooking. So how did its customers fall victim to *agona*? Remember that salmonella lives in the gut. No doubt *agona* was part of the natural gut flora of the fish off the coasts of Peru; it would do little harm there. After the hens began to eat the dried fish meal, *agona* found a new permanent home. No doubt the poultry was 'drawn' before being supplied but during that process the carcasses would be contaminated. It is likely that at the restaurant the meat was prepared using the same knives, surfaces and even utensils that were later used, without an obvious need for them to be cleaned, for those items on the menu which did not require cooking – the cabbage for coleslaw for example. It would be unreasonable to expect the cook to wash his hands after each bird had been prepared; and how many of us would be sufficiently knowledgeable to appreciate the need? Fortunately, this sequence of events is unlikely to lead to disastrous consequences in the home since salmonella need to be ingested in large numbers (by adults, that is), in the order of tens of thousands to be able to invade, a quantity which would in these circumstances only be achieved by repetitive enhancement. It is conceivable that a few organisms residing in the sauce of a coleslaw after its preparation would readily multiply at room temperature in a restaurant.

That is not the end of the *agona* story. The organism is now commonplace in pigs, on pig farms, abattoirs and in pork meat products; there is more than a suspicion that it is thriving through the recycling of waste products from animal husbandry back to animals. It has extended its geographical base; even the Iron Curtain has not been able to keep *agona* out. It has been fished out of the water and clearly thrives on land, like the seagulls we see in winter.

*

'By adults', in parenthesis above, was more than a hint that the situation is different in the young. It used to be a comforting thought that infection by salmonella could only come about if many organisms were swallowed. This view is no longer tenable: a small number of organisms, mild contamination that is, is all that is necessary to infect infants. How this came to light is yet another indication of the ramifications of salmonella activity.

There is an abnormality a few babies are born with: cystic fibrosis. Fortunately it is rare for it affects the lungs and other organs, and can prove fatal. One of the other organs is the pancreas with the result that it fails to secrete the digestive juice that organ is normally responsible for – the enzyme, pancreatin. Lack of pancreatin leads to malnutrition. To overcome this omission an extract of pancreatin is made from the pancreases of pigs and fed to an affected baby by mouth. In 1972 came the first reports of salmonella infection involving two such babies, not more than four and five months old; in view of the year this happened the organism had to be *agona*. One baby became a carrier; the other developed gastroenteritis and everybody at home became infected too.

The method used for the preparation of the pancreatin would not have permitted bacterial contamination in large numbers; moreover during its preparation, test samples were examined at frequent and regular intervals. So only the occasional organism must have slipped through the safety nets of the production procedures. Yet this was enough. Complete sterilisation was impossible since the pancreatin would have been destroyed in the process.

That incident was only the beginning; such was the degree of contamination of pigs' carcasses with other salmonella in the abattoirs, no doubt from organisms in the animals' guts, that on occasions between 1975 and 1977 it became impossible to provide uncontaminated pancreatin; yet such is the need for pancreatin in these babies that the risk of causing gastroenteritis had to be accepted.

As we grow up we acquire more protection through the increasing acidity of our stomach juices; so possibly, from childhood onwards, salmonella need to be present in overwhelming numbers to enable a few organisms to run the acid gauntlet and survive, and so get through into the intestine where theoretically only one or two bacteria can survive to multiply. But this depends to some extent upon what we eat. Another revealing epidemic developed in 1973 in Canada and the USA; again the search for the source was facilitated by the fact that the type of salmonella was very rare in those countries – the *eastbourne* variety. The trail led to a chocolate factory in Canada where the culprit was identified; *salmonella eastbourne* was being conveyed there by the cocoa beans which were probably contaminated when exposed to human and animal excreta during the process of harvesting, fermenting and drying of the beans in West Africa. Samples of the contaminated chocolate revealed no more than one thousand bacteria per pound. They probably escaped the acid bath through being protected by the fat in the chocolate.

If the thought that you may not be safe with a bar of chocolate makes you feel uneasy there is more to come, for through chocolate doubt has now been cast upon the concept that, in adults at least, penetration by salmonella through the acid barrier of the stomach is only successfully achieved in large numbers.

From April to September 1982 there began to appear in the UK a strain seldom if ever seen here, *salmonella napoli*: during that period there were over two hundred cases of dysentery reported due to this bacterium. Where did the organism come from and how did it get here? Hardly surprisingly, the source of *napoli* was in Italy; more so was the vehicle: chocolate. Tommy Junior and Rocky Junior bars were manufactured in northern Italy and sold cheaply in markets over here. A couple of enterprising bacteriologists working in a public health laboratory in Poole, Dorset, thought they would turn this misfortune to advantage. Bacteria cannot thrive and multiply in chocolate as they can in moist succulent juices like the sauce of a coleslaw. The organisms are simply locked in, lying quietly dormant in their solid surroundings, until released by digestion as from Pandora's box. All the two microbiologists had to do was to discover the number of bacteria embedded in a given quantity of chocolate, then work out from this figure and the number of bars eaten by patients in their neighbourhood the probable dose of organisms each received. They were fortunate as regards one patient, a boy of ten who had eaten one bar on each of two successive days, because both his mother and thirteen year old brother had also partaken of two bars, each in one day. Furthermore the brother, though symptom free, was found to be excreting *napoli*. From the case and the carrier it was an easy matter to work out that not more than about 50 bacteria were needed to start off dysentery.

By comparison, in the *eastbourne* epidemic evidence indicated that 1000 or so organisms may be all that is needed, whereas it had been thought that tens of thousands if not millions were required in an inoculum of salmonella to bring on dysentery. So attitudes are having to be revised, though some variation is to be expected between different members of the salmonella group; for bacteria vary in virulence, a characteristic which must in part reflect their ability to resist destruction in such an unfavourable milieu as the acidity of the stomach.

These incidents show how bacterial infections of the gut crop up where least expected. It is old hat that typhoid is conveyed by water and paratyphoid by milk but who would have expected to find another salmonella closely akin to these, lurking in dried yeast? What can be done in the face of the intensified farming necessary to provide us with an adequate food supply, involving practices which necessitate keeping animals and poultry confined in com-pounds at close quarters where their food and water may become contaminated by their own excreta. With meat, bone and fish meal being fed back to animals, the likelihood of infection increases, a vicious circle which the Danes long ago took steps to break by insisting upon sterilisation of feed containing animal ingredients. Once contamination has occurred in a herd, whether of poultry or pigs, it is difficult to eradicate; one farm rearing turkeys caused various epidemics of salmonella food poisoning in England over a period of eight years. How easy for salmonella to spread throughout flocks and herds, or be introduced by rodents and even birds. Seagulls provide a case in point; they have become landlubbers at least in the winter months. The danger from them lies not so much in what organisms they may be harbouring in their gut when they come off the sea – who knows, they might have *salmonella agona* – but in their habits when they arrive. They follow the plough, and that is no problem for as the plough turns the sod it is the grubs and the worms they are after. It is when they move away from the rural scene close to the sea, up estuaries to our large conurbations that the trouble begins. They become the scavengers at the local sewage works and the next moment join other water-loving birds on the inviting nearby stretches of water presented by the reservoirs. It is not difficult to see the potential health hazard in this, a potential which is growing as the behaviour of gulls continues to change and develop in this way.

*

And this is by no means the end of the sad story; there is the family of *shigella*. As they only infect man and the monkey it might be thought that shigella would not be a very serious competitor to salmonella. Since the shigellae exist only in the intestines of primates and few of us can boast of more than a nodding acquaintance with a monkey on trips to the zoo in days of our youth, it follows that we can only infect one another. Indeed this is only achieved when simple hygiene fails. But shigella has one considerable advantage over salmonella, which has to be swallowed in some number, in doses measured in thousands, for a few to get through the acidity of the stomach. Not so the shigellae; ten to one hundred will suffice to produce diarrhoea. So a shigella does not even need a nourishing pabulum like milk or food in which to multiply as salmonella sometimes does before it can be effective in its attack upon man.

From this it may be properly inferred that we can provide no natural barrier to shigella when it comes our way; the acid in the stomach is no bar to *shigella sonnei*, the commonest member of the breed. It only requires a slight faecal contamination of the fingers, such as might persist after a perfunctory ablution, to pass the organism from a carrier to a new victim; homosexuals are much at risk. Matters have become much worse where drainage is faulty so that sewage can contaminate water supply, or where the carrier happens to be a cook. Then an epidemic develops, as has been known to happen in the confines of a cruise ship or an airliner. An epidemic of bacillary dysentery of this nature today is unpleasant to say the least, but not as serious as when Dr Shiga first described this cause of diarrhoea at the end of the last century. That was in Japan and about a quarter of those affected died; but the organism was what was then known as Shiga's bacillus (*shigella dysenteriae*),

48

which for some inexplicable reason has given way to *shigella sonnei*, a less fatal strain. But bacteria move in a mysterious way; differing strains have their unpredictable ups and downs. *Shigella sonnei* has been on the up and up since between the two world wars; but warning of a more unpleasant future of greater violence comes from India and Central America where in recent epidemics *shigella dysenteriae* has again raised its ugly head.

*

Bacteria move in different ways their damage to achieve, some simply flourish in foodstuff, multiplying there and manufacturing poison. Staphylococci, which usually lurk on the skin where they may become responsible for pimples, boils and carbuncles, can do this. It is not difficult to imagine an infected finger contaminating food during the preparation of cakes, custards and pastries, where these bacteria find a nice sugary mixture to their liking, a culture medium in which they can flourish. The toxin they produce then soaks into the food, is swallowed and food poisoning results. Staphylococci are not uncommonly to blame for epidemics of diarrhoea and vomiting, for food handlers are not always aware of this danger from unhealed abrasions and cuts.

What is more, the routine medical examination of food handlers before they are employed is deemed unnecessary in the UK even by the Department of Health; sadly many are ill trained and unqualified, though officials known as environmental health officers are beginning to organise courses for cooks and their assistants.

The outcome of staphylococcal contamination is nothing like as serious as the effects of *clostridium botulinum*, which causes botulism and is hardly part of our story since it is associated with paralysis and not with diarrhoea. Nevertheless botulism is due to food poisoning and it is very fatal, so it is fortunate that it is also very rare; but like the staphylococcus this clostridium which poisons us when it succeeds in getting into food – usually a can of meat, sometimes of vegetables – does so by the poison it is able to elaborate there.

49

Other bacteria grow in the gut and develop their toxins there: cholera, and the coliform organisms (responsible for traveller's diarrhoea), while shigella and those salmonellae just discussed do so in part, but not wholly. The human salmonellae, that is those members of the species which live primarily in man's gut either as carriers or as a cause of typhoid or paratyphoid, by contrast invade the intestinal wall itself; shigellae are able to do both. Indeed, shigella can have two bites at the cherry: when it has got a hold in the small intestine it becomes effective by the local effect of its toxin which causes acute diarrhoea and vomiting shortly after infection has taken place. But this may sometimes be followed after two or three days by a change in symptoms to frequent bloody stools of small volume being passed after a wave of colic and with pain in the rectum. This change from the acute vomiting and diarrhoea of food poisoning to the symptoms of dysentery marks a change in attack not only in site, from the small intestine to the colon, but also in style, for in the large intestine the bacteria penetrate the mucosal cells, the cells of the lining epithelium that is, and actually reproduce there, rather than remain outside the tissue in the hollow of the gut as they do in the jejunum. That second phase is in effect a colitis, a specific form of colitis – specific because its cause is known, recognisable and recognised. Once within the epithelial cell, it seems likely that the bacteria can produce another poison which reacts against the tiny structures known as organelles to be seen within the cell sap (cytoplasm) and responsible for its function: but this still remains a matter of speculation.

The salmonellae responsible for typhoid and paratyphoid, although they similarly gain access to the interstices of individual mucosal cells, are less destructive. This may be an indication of a different toxic system; certainly the pattern of the illness as it develops is very different in typhoid, which starts with a week or so of headache, abdominal pain and increasing fever to be followed in the second week by diarrhoea which lacks one aspect of colitis, bloody stools, because the mucosa does not become ulcerated in the way that it does in shigellosis. However, the passage of blood and nothing but blood in the third week of the illness, in contrast to a diarrhoeic stool of fluid faeces contaminated with blood, is an alarming, spectacular and dangerous development of untreated typhoid. It occurs because lymph glands, incorporated within the colon wall, particularly in the further reaches of the small intestine (the ileum), break down and ulcerate.

*

There is one other form of dysentery: *entamoeba histolytica* is a parasite comprising only one cell, technically a protozoon, with a liking for human red blood cells. Unlike the malarial parasite, which has a similar penchant, it obtains them by burrowing from the lumen of the large bowel into the mucosa undermining its epithelial cover and so ulcerating that surface. The amoeba is passed from man to man through contaminated food and drink, cold drinks in particular, and is common where sanitation and hygiene are poor. Nicely encapsulated in an inert cyst-like form, which gives it a protective skin, the amoeba moves down the gut unharmed until it reaches the large bowel where it blossoms forth into a mobile cell much larger than a bacterium, easily seen under the low power magnification of a microscope if the circumstances of its environment there are right. If it is comfortably moist and warm, it may be seen on the rampage after red blood cells, moving remarkably adroitly by simply flowing in the right direction and then pouring itself around its quarry engulfing and digesting it. The ulceration it causes in gaining access to its needs in the bowel is often of sufficient severity to cause dysentery so that bloody diarrhoea ensues; the mucosa becoming generally inflamed to produce another specific form of colitis.

*

For food poisoning, treatment is frequently a matter of *laissez-fair*; for dysentery it is more active. The choice lies between whether or not to use antibiotic drugs. A good example of the dilemma is to be found in the salmonellae; food poisining brought about by any of the multifarious forms of salmonella, though sharp and unpleasant, in

51

effect is short-lived. Except in the unusual case, there is no evidence that antibiotic drugs substantially relieve the duration or symptoms of the illness; indeed there is evidence that their use may prolong an attack of gastroenteritis. Moreover there is always the concern that the drug will eliminate less harmful organisms ordinarily inhabiting the colon competing with the abnormal ones. An antibiotic can render the circumstances more favourable for the salmonella in more ways than one, for it may encourage antibiotic-resistant forms to develop. As with traveller's diarrhoea so in food poisoning; emphasis is laid upon easing the discomfort and the diarrhoea, and by the same means.

But typhoid is a different matter; here the salmonella invade to create an infection of the intestines, but not just the intestines, since they have the habit of getting into the blood to be spread far and wide and arriving at a destination of their choice such as the gall bladder and kidney, settling there. From the first of these two organs the organisms may continue to be passed into the gut and excreted long after the illness has subsided, so turning a patient into a carrier; from the second into the urine with a similar outcome. So there are several reasons for wishing to eradicate *salmonella typhi* and its half brother *paratyphi*: typhoid is a serious illness with a septicaemic phase which may cause the patient to die, and the disease might be spread into an epidemic by a carrier. Once a carrier state has been achieved the bacteria are difficult to eliminate by antibiotics, so that the organ in which the bacteria reside needs to be removed if it can be spared; the gall bladder is dispensible, the kidneys are not.

Shigellosis falls into both categories. No more than symptomatic treatment is needed for gastroenteritis, but on the first sign of dysentery developing an antibiotic is likely to be prescribed though the choice is hampered by the ability of shigella to take on protective plasmid raincoats.

There is no therapeutic dilemma as regards intestinal parasites whether they be small simple cells like amoebae or large and complex structures like worms. We possess no immunity to them, nor are we capable of developing it. So the position is not comparable with bacterial invasion. Diarrhoea due to amoebiasis or giardiasis (chapter 1) is treated forthwith once the cause is known; there are special and effective drugs with which to do so. Intestinal worms are seldom a cause of diarrhoea and need not concern us here other than to say that they too have to be eliminated by appropriate drugs because of the anaemia and malnutrition they cause.

4 Persistent trouble in the bowel

Colitis is a word used to denote changes brought about by inflammation in the colon; there are many ways in which such inflammation comes about, most of which are difficult to distinguish from one another either from looking at the bowel with the naked eye or with the aid of a microscope, for inflammation is a general response brought into play by very complex mechanisms. A look down a microscope at a suitably prepared piece of inflamed colon would reveal an invasion of cells within the depth of the mucosa itself, in the supporting tissue of indeterminate architecture which lies between the mucosal epithelial cells facing the inside of the colon (the lumen) and the muscle layers which form the outer sheath. In the past this area has been named rather dismissively as connective-tissue, or stroma, no doubt because it seemed to be of minor importance in terms of function when compared with the epithelium on the one side and the muscle on the other, the stroma merely separating the two in a purely structural way. These appellations were assigned to this area when little or nothing was known about inflammatory cells and their function. Only very recently have we begun to appreciate what these cells in the connective tissue are capable of and how they achieve what they have to do. This connective tissue area is as important in its way as is the epithelium which covers it; it is a power house in which inflammatory cells are produced, many for local use some being dispatched to be set to work elsewhere in the body.

What are these cells? To avoid going into too great detail, they may be summarised as forming a group of which each member possesses a different ability, their common purpose being protection. They are the same as white blood cells, so called because a smear of blood on a microscope slide will show, on the one hand, red cells capable of carrying oxygen around the body by virtue of the red pigment, haemoglobin, which they contain, and on the other and in less profusion more opaque cells without a hint of pigment and, unlike the red cells, containing nuclei. These nuclei are the stamp, as it were, of their living identity, the proof that they do not just exist but are capable of purposeful controlled activity and reproduction, which the red blood cells are not. Red cells have one function and one only: to carry oxygen. They are being constantly poured out by their nucleated progenitors from the core of the bones into the blood stream. After about three weeks the wear and tear of squeezing through the tiny tubes of the microcapillaries where they impart their oxygen to the surrounding tissues, begins to tell upon their flexible mantles – the ageing red cell is then withdrawn from circulation and its capsule broken open so that the tiny dose of haemoglobin can be released and reprocessed in order to provide fresh new unadulterated haemoglobin for the next lot of red cells being formed in the bone marrow.

For the white cells and inflammatory cells anywhere in the body the situation is rather different. They have to cope with any invasive trouble. Particularly is this so in the colon, teeming as it is with bacteria, some of which can turn nasty. All too easy for a harmful bacterium or its toxin to gain access through a surface which allows absorption, as in the colon; here in contrast to the skin, which is watertight, cells of the epithelium are put together to allow water at least to pass through.

There is a group of inflammatory cells which have the ability to engulf particulate matter, flowing around their prey as some amoebae do around red blood cells. Their quarry may be bacteria, parasites or small particles of material foreign to the body; or like carrion crows they can home in on the debris of dead cells, scavenging and cleaning up the mess. Another group of cells has a more sophisticated task: to manufacture chemicals to counteract the toxins which emanate from bacteria, and antidotes to the organisms themselves – to any antigen, in fact; a term which covers anything from inert chemicals like bacterial poison to living protein such as viruses or bacteria. There is no telling where the next blow may come from, nor what it will be or what form it may take. So the inflammatory cells have to be endowed with the capability of analysing a noxious substance, the flexibility to match it with the appropriate antidote and the capacity to manufacture sufficient of that antidote from the protein material at their disposal in the blood stream. The result is an immunoglobulin. The neutralisation thus achieved is a physical process involving the locking of one chemical molecule onto another, in the same way that two adjacent pieces of a jigsaw puzzle fit decisively in the right place and will not fit if incorrectly placed.

Every molecule has its own distinctive individual shape so each antigen has to be matched with its own special antibody which alone will fit it, like the tumblers of a lock will match one key. It is inconceivable that the body could carry around with it a compendium of antibodies sufficient to meet all possible contingencies likely to be encountered in a lifetime; think of the load this would entail and the prescience it would require. A vast number of immune complexes – at its simplest, the interactions of antigen with antibody – have to be formed during a lifetime from a set of immunoglobulins but nowhere more than in the colon, where the process is being conducted continuously during health, more so during disease, and particularly in colitis. Sometimes the process overreaches itself and leads to disease on its own account; the immune complex itself becomes a cause for further inflammation when lymphocytes, another member of the inflammatory cell group, become engaged. But more of that anon.

The other aspects of inflammation which catch the eye are in a sense incidental. There is much engorgement with blood, for the needs of the situation demand improved blood supply – of white cells in particular and their requirements. Moreover in certain forms of infection there is an attempt to contain the situation by enclosing it; this being achieved by creating a *cordon sanitaire* of blood clot – another reason for the increased blood supply. An abscess is the outcome and the process applies particularly to staphylococcal skin infections, boils for example, but would not be evident in the colon, for good reason. There in the mucosa the initial stages of the inflammatory process are not incompatible with health. Indeed the appearances of mild inflammatory change is part of the normal activity to maintain health, an indication that that tissue is carrying out its function of protection satisfactorily as the second line of defence against the bacteria banging at the door; the first being the rather leaky barrier of epithelial cells, leaky because of the fluid fluxes which have to flow between them and indeed the particulate matter in molecular form which has to cross the cytoplasmic territory of their cells. If clotting were part of this interplay it would defeat the purpose, which is to cope with chance bacterial trespass without causing a general disturbance; clotting would constitute a major change in the cellular status quo.

It is impossible to say from these microscopic appearances at what juncture the boundaries of normality have been transgressed. A markedly increased number of inflammatory cells is suggestive. Incontrovertible signs of abnormality are to be seen elsewhere; those sensitive epithelial cells begin to look sick, either distorted with swelling or actually beginning to separate away from the connective tissue which supports them. Thus ulceration begins.

At regular intervals along the surface of the mucosa the sheet of epithelium dips into the mucosal substance to form simple glands. Mention of these 'crypts' has already been made in relation to the small intestine and its function (chapter 1). Down in the colon they are simpler in form as befits their function there, since digestive enzymes are not needed at this level, mucus being the only substance required – as far as we know. As the cells at the mouth of a glandular crypt become swollen so the tubular central cavity tends to get blocked off from the bowel lumen into which it should be passing the mucus its cells are secreting. In effect a microscopic cyst is formed; but rather more than that for the retained contents become infected, a lot of white cells collect there and die, and the mini-cyst has become a mini-abscess, albeit different in creation from the staphylococcal abscess. As the inflammation becomes more severe the surface of the mucosa is torn away to a level deeper than the orifices of these glands when some crypt abscesses will be exposed and will drain away.

Abscesses have a tendency to burst out from their confines. They sometimes have to be lanced and drained, not only to relieve painful swelling but also to prevent rupture in the wrong direction, which could be dangerous. Clearly it is inconceivable that these tiny crypt abscesses could be drained in this way, yet they have the same capacity to burst out in an uncontrolled fashion and they do so along paths of least resistance. Rupture tends to occur into the connective tissue alongside; the pus then pours into another plane where it is directed sideways.

That plane in the interstices of the bowel wall is brought about by a structure which has not yet been mentioned. Besides the layers of circular and longitudinal muscle which accomplish the transport of its contents down the gut by the various manoeuvres of peristalsis, there is a thinner hardly perceptible layer of muscle which is placed between the embedded ends of the glands, their apices, and the muscles just referred to. In the duodenum and upper jejunum where the demand upon the glands to produce enzymes is such that they need to extend further, this is achieved by branching and by extension through the muscularis mucosae, as the thin muscle is called, into the area beyond, which we identify as the submucosa. But in the large bowel the crypts, which are small and unbranched, have no need to penetrate into the submucosa.

57

We really know little about the function of this space other than what can be deduced from the microscopic appearances. It is obviously a substation for blood vessels, a network arising from the main arteries when they reach the gut, from which smaller vessels run inwards to supply the needs of the mucosa itself while rather fewer pass backwards to feed the muscle wall. The equally important veins follow the same course but the blood they contain flows in the opposite direction. One other clearly discernible feature in the submucosal area is the congregation of lymph cells in what are described as follicles. Less easily discernible are the intercommunicating mesh of specialised nerves in plexuses which automatically control intestinal movement without our having to be aware of the activity.

The muscularis mucosae has no place in our story of the flux other than as a line of demarcation, a little landmark which enables mucosa to be differentiated from submucosa, of some importance in the differentiation of ulcerative colitis from Crohn's disease, and as a mark against which may be gauged the depth of ulceration when it occurs in the large bowel. Of its function there is no more to say than that by contracting it is able to fold the mucosa into the gut lumen like the bellows of an accordion, so as to increase the exposure of gut contents to the area of absorption.

*

The manner in which various tissues react can present a pattern of abnormality from which it may be possible to identify the cause. The colitis induced by the amoeba *entamoeba histolytica* is usually quite distinctive. Ulcers are clearly to be seen by the naked eye, the edges appearing to be undermined, as indeed they are; for once through the epithelial layer the parasites nibble away sideways underneath it. An inflammatory reaction precedes them so that the edges of the ulcers seen through a microscope or a colonoscope may be marked with a reddened halo. The cause is confirmed by seeing the amoebae either in a piece of tissue removed from the edge of the ulcer to be examined under the microscope, or by catching one or two of the parasites on a small swab designed for the purpose. But amoebiasis does not always take on this recognisable pattern; in the Middle East where the condition is rife, and rarely in the UK, it can present in an acute form indistinguishable from severe ulcerative colitis. Unless the possibility is borne in mind and parasites are looked for in the stools of such cases the diagnosis can go by default with dire consequences.

It is a different matter with ulcerative colitis; here is a disease of no recognisable cause and its appearance presents no distinctive hallmark. Looking at an affected bowel it is obvious that the epithelial surface has been damaged and perhaps lost, for it looks raw in the same way that eczema or a badly abraded skin does. There is general ulceration though within the affected area there are no distinct ulcers outlined by way of contrast with intervening patches of intact epithelium. This is not to say that the large bowel is always affected in its entirety; more often only a part of its length is involved; but however limited the condition the rectum is always included. This, at one time, caused misunderstanding and doctors propounded that the condition started in the rectum; of this there is no evidence only that it may be confined to that region. Put another way: however extensive or limited the area of large bowel affected by the disease, the rectum is always included.

*

Ulcerative colitis is unpredictable in a number of ways: in severity, in duration of attacks and as regards the length of intestine that may become involved. It has a distinctive feature; it is confined to the large intestine. Reflecting the changes which take place in the tissue it frequently starts with the appearance of blood in the motions as the bowel surface becomes raw and starts to ooze; and pain is often a feature of the first attack, in the form of colic. After two or three days, diarrhoea begins; the colic then ceases and does not return even in further attacks. Diarrhoea is severe in both respects: the bowels open frequently, sometimes as often as every hour, and the stool is fluid. Another point: it is very common for a patient with ulcerative colitis to be woken in the night by the need to evacuate the bowel.

But though the constancy of the way the illness starts may be distinctive, it does not distinguish ulcerative colitis from other causes of colitis. So the diagnosis is first made by establishing that active inflammation is present in the large bowel, and this is achieved very simply by looking through a sigmoidoscope and taking a biopsy sample for study under the microscope. X-ray pictures using the radio-opaque material, barium sulphate, as an enema show up the mucosal outline and the general configuration of the bowel; in ulcerative colitis the normal segmental pattern tends to be lost leaving a straightened tube. But any of the specific causes of diarrhoea, in particular the dysenteries, might be responsible so they have to be excluded. In one respect the course of the disorder gives a clue; the fact that diarrhoea has persisted for many days if not weeks makes an infective cause unlikely since the effects of food poisoning are relatively short lived and the duration of the dysenteries are circumscribed. But as in all matters medical there are seldom clear cut distinctions, so in diarrhoeic disorders there are all shades of severity – an identifiable dysentery, as caused by *campylobacter* for example, may occasionally persist. Thus the symptoms of one condition can coincide with or overlap another. So another necessity on the way to the diagnosis of ulcerative colitis is the exclusion by the bacteriological laboratory of the presence of known bacteria and parasites from the stools. In effect the diagnosis is made by default, through the fact that no recognisable cause can be demonstrated.

A distressing feature of ulcerative colitis is its predelic-tion for the young; it most commonly develops between the ages of twenty and thirty, is by no means rare before twenty and sometimes starts in childhood. The youngest patient I have ever had to treat was a baby under a year old, but that *was* an exception.

We must not lose sight of the fact that here is an un-common condition. Its incidence is about six new cases diagnosed in 100,000 persons in the UK population each year. This figure in isolation is perhaps not very compre-hensible, but to put it in perspective the incidence of bowel cancer is 24 men and 31 women each year in a population of 100,000. The incidence of ulcerative colitis is much the same elsewhere in the world where such statistics can be reasonably assessed – Scandinavia and USA for example – though it appears to be lower by half in Israel.

Another statistic by which the rarity or otherwise of a disease is measured is its prevalence, which is a way of stating how many sufferers may be found at any one time, as opposed to how many new cases develop each year. This works out at anything from 40 to 80 per 100,000 people – not very many cases. These two statistics, incidence and prevalence, indicate different aspects in the natural history of a disease. The two do not go hand in hand. Increase in frequency carries the obvious implication that the disease is actually on the increase; there is no evidence that this is occurring with ulcerative colitis. As far as we know (there is no exactitude in population statistics) the incidence of six per 100,000 has remained the same since it was first disclosed in 1960 by doctors working in Oxford. Clearly the prevalence of a condition would fall, even when the incidence remained unchanged, if therapy became more effective through a specific treatment being found, or contrariwise if the death rate increased. There has been no evidence of either.

Another feature in what might be termed the natural history of the disease is the fact that it is more common in women, by about two to one. There was a time when it was thought to be a disease virtually of whites, in the western world and temperate climates at that. I can recall the *obiter dicta* of almost half a century ago when it was thought that ulcerative colitis was to be found in those the Americans call caucasian (their term for someone ethnically white) in the northern states, but was said to be rare in the extreme in the southern states such as Mississippi, Louisiana and Alabama. Now we know this is not so; possibly dysentery was so much more rife then in the southern states that it masked ulcerative colitis. Likewise the belief that ulcerative colitis was not to be seen on the Indian continent has subsequently been discredited. What we cannot tell is the

61

incidence in such areas because of the difficulty of register-
ing and documenting cases there. For all we know it may be
as common in India, Africa and Asia as the West, and in
blacks as whites. There is one small piece of evidence,
however, of ethnic predilection, it is slightly but statistically
commoner in Jews – but outside Israel it would seem!

The observation has already been made that ulcerative
colitis is unpredictable in several ways; it may start mildly
or with great severity. This reflects both the depth and
extent to which the large intestine is affected. It takes little
imagination to see that the deeper the disease bites into the
mucosa and the wider the area over which it does so, the
greater will be the severity of the diarrhoea. The capacity of
the colon to absorb fluid will be reduced the greater the area
of involvement. In addition more of the body's fluid – tissue
fluid and serum from the blood – will leach out, the wider
and deeper the ulcers.

Such is the nature of ulcerative colitis that what began as
mild disease may continue so over many years, either
continuously or in intermittent attacks. Moreover the re-
missions punctuating these periods of illness are variable
and of unforseeable duration. So it would be wrong to
suppose that once the condition has occurred a natural
progression takes hold, of ever increasing damage and
severity. There are patients who get it so mildly that they
are virtually not disabled and remain in this state for the
rest of their lives over periods of thirty to forty years or
more; though this is unusual and carries with it a specially
sinister danger which will be considered shortly.

It is important to clarify this point before pursuing
further how the disease may progress from the early stages
of ulceration, in order to avoid the false impression that one
stage of abnormality leads automatically to the next, in ever
increasing stages of severity. Moreover although healing
occurs when an attack ends and to all intents and purposes
the microscopic appearances of the gut lining look normal
again (though this is not always the case), something is
nevertheless incomplete and healing must in some way be
imperfect. When a further relapse develops the same area

of the bowel is always affected; not infrequently new sites are included. In addition, during remission when the patient is free of symptoms and examination through a sigmoidoscope shows no ulceration, an x-ray will often reveal persistence of an unusual, straight, tubular appearance in the area of the bowel that was involved, an appearance which arises not from any change in the mucosa but from alteration in the tone of the muscle of the colon.

One isolated attack of bloody diarrhoea would not constitute ulcerative colitis; it is a disease of recurrence, so once the changes have taken place a trigger has been set for further attacks of diarrhoea in the future. Conversely it is not a disease which can be cured; the best we can achieve is to bring an attack under control and once remission has been obtained endeavour to prolong this for as long as possible. To say that ulcerative colitis is an incurable disease would be strictly true; but that term has a strong emotive meaning inevitably linked to cancer with all its implications of fatality. Ulcerative colitis can prove fatal, but only when serious complications have supervened. The situation is like duodenal ulcer, which everyone knows as a common condition causing indigestion. Duodenal ulcer cannot be cured; though the ulcer may heal between episodes of indigestion it is always prone to break down again – unless, of course, it has been removed. Duodenal ulcer, too, can prove fatal but so rarely as to induce none of the fear we associate with the incurability and fatality of cancer; the situation is not dissimilar in ulcerative colitis.

A remission develops in concert with healing of the mucosa, as epithelial cells reassert themselves and regain lost ground across the inflamed ulcerated connective tissue. The process is almost identical with what happens on the skin. Ulceration there whether from injury such as abrasion, burn or some other cause heals from the edge inwards until the gap is closed; we have all seen this happen in ourselves. Those epithelial cells of the skin, still alive and intact at the edges of the ulcer, multiply to furnish a sheet of cells which begin to provide cover as infection in the ulcer begins to subside. Moreover, if the ulcer has not

63

penetrated too far into the depths of the skin, what is left of the hair follicles and ducts of the sweat glands will provide further sources from which epithelial replacement can take place, as though the ulcer base had been peppered with tiny active seedlings. So it is in the colon: mucosal epithelium is regenerated from the edges of the affected areas and, more importantly, from the many nests of cells, the remains of attenuated glands; for these crypts dip into the substance of the mucosa and are not completely obliterated unless the mucosa is destroyed in its full depth. The remnants of these glands are therefore of the greatest importance when it comes to healing; indeed without them it will not be complete for it would be imposssible to cover from the edges alone areas as extensive as those exposed by ulcerative colitis.

Healing thus achieved will only restore normal mucosal architecture when the initial damage has been light. Even then abnormality persists in some invisible way, leaving a fragile mucosa. Once the epithelial veil has been torn apart it is a matter of chance how much of the underlying supporting structure is lost. In mild disease this is slight and of little consequence; when healing takes place the thickness of the mucosa has been maintained so that all can be restored to the *status quo ante*. It is usual, however, for loss to occur beyond the epithelium to variable depth. The supporting tissue below the epithelium is not regained so that when epithelial coverage takes place the mucosa may be a shadow of its former self, thin with short squat glands. Indeed the epithelial cells may not acquire their full stature; instead of being rectangles stood on end (columnar) they appear rectangular (cuboid). The new lining is weak and, no doubt, more prone than before to breakdown like those longstanding scars which cover healed chronic ulcers of the leg or extensive burns.

In addition the glandular crypts may contribute to the instability of the repaired mucosa. Reference has already been made to the manner in which some crypts are turned into micro-abscesses as a result of the ducts which drain them becoming blocked. Not every crypt abscess develops to the point where it either bursts into the bowel lumen or reversely into the wall itself to develop further there as an intramural abscess; some remain modest in size, and still confined within the encysted shell which follows distension of the small gland by the inflammatory exudate it now contains. So it may be when remission catches up with a crypt abscess; so it may remain when the epithelium closes over to restore continuity of the mucosal lining once more. Much of the purulent content of the micro-abscess may become absorbed as quiescence falls upon the inflammatory scene; nevertheless the abnormality remains, further to sap the integrity of the mucosa and increase its susceptibility to future attack.

The mucosa is now less able to undertake its normal function; it is weakened in its role of keeping at bay those organisms teeming in the large bowel lumen. The nice balance maintained by the inflammatory cells is disturbed not only because the thickness of the mucosa and numbers of defensive cells have been reduced, but also because the apparently burnt out micro-abscesses may flare again into activity through inflammation close by and so explode, to the destruction of the tissue around and epithelium above. Thus the attenuated, abnormal mucosa, although apparently healed in the sense that it is not ulcerated, can break down too readily when encountering challenges which would cause no disturbance in normal circumstances, and so fall once more from grace to recrudescence. Another attack of bloody diarrhoea is then set in motion; the mucosa will be damaged further as infection from the gut organisms gain easy access once more; it will probably take longer before remission is achieved; the quiescent mucosa thereafter will be even less stable; the period of the next remission is likely to be shorter, if indeed a full remission is gained at all. Some patients even have to contend with persistent diarrhoea which relents only to the extent that the frequency of stool varies between moments of improvement and periods of exacerbation.

*

All of us have suffered diarrhoea at some occasion in our lives; all of us have suffered the uncertainty, the indignity and the incapacity which follows in its train. The episodes we have had to put up with, due to food poisoning or viral infections, have been short lived in comparison with what patients with ulcerative colitis have to endure. Whereas we may have been incapacitated for two or three days at the most, even a brief attack of ulcerative colitis is likely to persist for as many months. It is not difficult to imagine the mental stress such a patient is subjected to, nor the besetting problems of daily living. Unless the condition is mild at the outset, he or she will almost certainly take to his or her bed (since the condition is commoner in women I shall use the female gender) in the expectation that the overriding symptom of diarrhoea which follows the initial day or two of pain and the passage of blood with an otherwise normal stool, will shortly subside. But the malaise and fever continue to linger longer than expected; the condition may get worse, in which circumstance she will probably be admitted to hospital, not infrequently to what used to be known as a fever or isolation hospital, but more probably into a bed on what is now called a communicable diseases unit, in order that a specific contagious dysentery may first be excluded. Or to a bed in a general ward.

Ironically the situation may be less easy when the symptoms are less severe; the patient remains at home and has to learn to contend with the problems posed there. As the diarrhoea abates she begins to return to normal life. This is not difficult to achieve in a full remission; only the general weakness which follows recumbancy and the debility induced by the illness itself has to be overcome. But the diarrhoea may not fully subside. It only has to persist in a relatively minor way to call for considerable adjustment. Though the bowels may open four or five times a day, as often as not there is an urgency in the desire to pass a motion, a precipitancy which brooks no denial. The housewife doing her shopping may have to plan her route according to where she knows toilets exist and relief can be obtained. A boy at school knows that uncontrollable incontinent disaster is only too possible playing football on a cold afternoon. The breadwinner is concerned as to whether he can reach the desk at his office or the bench at work before intolerable nature calls.

Contending with the daily round is tiring enough; in addition there are the effects of anaemia. At the stage when the acuteness of the condition wanes and the frequency of bowel action diminishes it may even appear that blood is no longer being passed. Nevertheless with persistent ulceration it is inevitable that some blood continues to be lost though insufficient in quantity to be evident or obvious. Such a continuous blood loss is to some extent compensated for; the blood-forming organs increase their turnover. One of the limiting factors in this process is the iron which is needed to produce haemoglobin, the chemical carried round the body in the red blood cells. Haemoglobin has the ability to take up oxygen in the lungs and release it where it is needed in the tissues; iron is an essential part of haemoglobin and cannot be replaced by any other element more readily available in the body such as sodium or potassium. Moreover iron is not easily absorbed from the gut even in normal circumstances; for this reason it is conserved when ageing red blood cells wear out and is passed back to the bone marrow to be used again in the formation of more haemoglobin. A constant loss of blood may exceed the ability of the body to absorb and process iron in quantities sufficient to replace the unremitting wastage. Hence the anaemia. Enough red cells may be there but with each containing too little haemoglobin, though under these circumstances the number of red cells usually falls short of the normal complement. Tiredness is a paramount feature of chronic anaemia due to iron deficiency, rather than shortness of breath as might be expected though this would become evident sooner than usual on physical exertion. The anaemic patient lacks energy.

*

The patient with chronic disease learns to adapt, even to endure the privations of her circumstances. Her condition and the straits she finds herself in can persist for ten, fifteen, twenty years or even more, until she is no longer cognisant of the meaning and positive sensation of good health.

For others the course of the disease changes rapidly for the worse until a serious and dangerous situation is reached. This can happen at the very outset or at any time later, another manifestation of the unpredictability of ulcerative colitis. In a man or woman whose affliction has for many years remained slight the disease may unexpectedly change from mild abnormality to alarming deterioration and the condition become one of emergency overnight.

The disintegrative process which accounts for this is fortunately rare – not more than five to ten per cent of all cases reach this stage. What happens is a progression of the destructive process already described. No doubt those crypt abscesses play a part by spreading out within the interstices of the bowel wall as intramural abscesses deep in the muscularis mucosae. The layers of mucosa lining the lumen at a superficial level are lifted away by this undermining process to leave the outer muscle zone devoid of any mucosal protection, exposed to the putrescent contents of the intestine. Already the submucosal area occupied by the communication system which controls the activity of the two groups of muscle has been transgressed, rendering those nerve plexuses incompetent if not completely inert. Now the circular muscle begins to break up as its constituent fibres are infiltrated by inflammation.

These two events spell disaster. The colon begins to give way under the tension of the gases it contains and the weight of the fluid contents which have now become stagnant in the more dependent areas. What is left of the colonic wall begins to perforate either directly into the peritoneal cavity so that the most serious form of peritonitis ensues, or it gives way in a less immediately disastrous manner. The hole is plugged by whatever may lie adjacent to it, usually by small intestine becoming stuck on to the colon all around the area of penetration – an act, it almost seems, of defence to limit peritoneal contamination as far as possible.

It is ironic that in this situation of acute colonic dilatation diarrhoea is suddenly alleviated. Bowel activity ceases not because its contents have poured into the abdominal cavity;

it stops before that can happen because the colon becomes inert, paralysed if you like, and cannot shift its contents onwards – a phenomenon which has been known to put the unwary or inexperienced doctor or nurse off their guard. On enquiring after such a patient I have often been assured by ward staff that there has been an improvement, on the evidence of cessation of the bowel motions. But one glance at a patient in these circumstances reveals abdominal distention as an outward and visible sign of the inner colonic distension.

Colonic dilatation represents a grave turn for the worse; even if perforation is avoided the risk of dying during this acute, severe deterioration is not less than fifty per cent. Though the half who survive do overcome the immediate dangers, the bowel is now so disordered that its removal is obligatory. The overwhelming nature of this development is only a reflection of a train of events associated with the breakdown of any form of protection within the bowel against its contents, and the severe biochemical disturbance which ensues.

Infection becomes all pervading; where the colon lies anatomically in direct contact with the wall of the abdominal cavity, that is in the flanks, infection can spread directly into the body and may provoke septicaemia, when bacteria not only gain access to the blood but thrive and multiply there. This is all the more likely when the colonic wall becomes completely eroded, as may happen. Meanwhile bacteria and toxins pour from the gut into the vital venous system which transports fluid and the results of digestion to the liver. Since the liver is both the storehouse for our nutritional needs and the powerhouse where much protein, in particular albumin, is put together, this bacteraemia soon begins to restrict and inhibit essential and vital functions. The liver starts to look sick, the cells contained in its pentagonal lobules showing a fatty change which indicates their imminent demise, while around the venous supply system lying between the lobules inflammation is all too evident. Jaundice may follow.

By this time lack of appetite, liver damage and failure of

intestinal function have conspired together to cause gross loss of weight, so much so that the patient may be reduced to skin and bone resembling the starved inmate of a concentration camp.

Chemical changes are equally extreme. Not only is the ability to absorb fluid impaired through loss of the absorptive power of the colonic mucosa, but much of the fluid within the body drains away continuously into the gut to contribute to the liquid stools. A curious contradiction develops; the body starts to dry out while at the same time beginning to display oedema, a paradoxical situation since oedema represents an abnormal collection of fluid. The paradox comes about in this way: while cells throughout the body are being deprived of the fluid they need within their cell sap, fluid is collecting in the spaces between the tissues. This is the outcome of a shortage of albumin, the protein in the serum of the blood responsible for retaining water there by osmosis. The blood albumin is constantly being drained away through the ulcerated colon; furthermore its replacement is denied by the disability in the liver.

Moreover another fundamental biochemical disturbance takes place; so much of the body's salt is lost in the fluid which drains away that the sodium ions it provides cannot be replaced: with the result that hydrogen ions, being the only cations readily to hand, begin to be employed in chemical reactions involving electrolytic exchange. The substitution of hydrogen for sodium creates a shift towards acidity within the cells. Since the whole bodily milieu is designed to remain neutral in order to accommodate the innumerable physiochemical reactions at cellular level, the smallest change towards acidity or alkalinity is a very serious matter because the reactions which contribute to viability are thereby inhibited. Small wonder then that with the considerable biochemical embarrassments brought about by this advanced stage of the illness the danger should be so great and death so likely to occur.

*

Let us turn away from this gloomy scene of acute chaos to consider more insidious implications which develop in the disease even in the milder form. Trouble may break out at sites in the body remote from the gut in unexpected ways. Fortunately these complications are uncommon, affecting no more than a tenth to a twentieth of those afflicted with ulcerative colitis. Eczema may begin to disfigure the skin, inflammation affect the eye in the form of iritis, and arthritis present with painful swelling at a knee, ankle, shoulder or hip – any of the larger joints in fact. All are probably secondary phenomena, immunological responses to the creation of abnormal immune compounds resulting from sensitisation by bacteria from the gut, or indeed any other protein element therein which could act as an antigen. Such antigenic sensitisation is facilitated by ulceration since this permits access of 'foreign' protein to the tissues and sets in train complex immune response. It is probably significant that when the large bowel is removed from a patient with one of these complications, arthritis, eczema or eye troubles subside almost overnight, presumably because the faulty immune system developing within the colon has been removed.

Jaundice is not only observed in the acute severe phase of ulcerative colitis; in the chronic condition of longer standing it is the outward and visible sign that cirrhosis is developing, or a very rare complication which causes the pipes which drain bile away from the liver to become inflamed.

The most serious development is the most insidious – cancer. For many years there was doubt as to whether cancer of the colon is a special hazard for the ulcerative colitis patient. About twenty years ago sufficient evidence was eventually forthcoming to establish that indeed colonic cancer is a special risk for those who have suffered from the condition for a long time. After ten years the risk becomes appreciable and increases as time passes. Its insidiousness arises from two features, the first being the long period that ulcerative colitis persists before malignant change develops. Inevitably this means that cancer is seen in milder cases of the disease, for when more severe the colon is likely to have been removed at an earlier stage before the

71

slow process of degeneration in the epithelial cells can become cancer. In addition, for patients who for many years have put up with recurrent attacks of bloody diarrhoea, no tocsin sounds to warn them that something further is amiss; for those precise symptoms, blood in the stools with or without diarrhoea, are what ordinarily alerts the non-colitic individual to the presence of cancer in the bowel.

The masking of the onset of cancer in ulcerative colitis has caused much difficulty in management of the long-standing case, for though abdominal pain may return with cancer, for the first time since the onset of ulcerative colitis, it is a late symptom, indicating advanced growth. To undertake barium x-rays at routine intervals in order to detect malignant change is impracticable for a number of reasons not least of which is the fact that cancer in ulcerative colitis not infrequently develops in a way which does not show up as a recognisable tumour. Should a patient, therefore, be advised to have the bowel removed on the sole basis that cancer might develop because ulcerative colitis has persisted for over ten years? The answer to this is made easier for both patient and doctor when other complications intervene, such as those just discussed; if not the decision can cause much heart searching.

Two developments have now relieved us of the uncertainty which gave rise to this difficult decision. The first was the realisation that where cancer develops, a distortion of both the mucosal architecture and the cells precedes it in a manner that is recognisable and different both from the distortion expected to follow the simple healing of ulceration and from the quiescence following inflammation. This change can sometimes be observed by the naked eye but it is most often brought to light in a biopsy sample taken through a sigmoidoscope.

One problem has remained: the precancerous distortion is patchy and though it may be present somewhere to incriminate the large bowel, this may not be in the area encompassed by a sigmoidoscope, the range of which is limited to 20 to 25 cms from the anus, since conventional optical systems demand direct lines of vision. Now that we have fibre optics at our disposal we can see round corners – through a flexible endoscope. The modern colonoscope enables the whole of the large intestine to be scanned from the anus backwards and it is possible to take samples of the mucosa at any level for microscopic examination, in particular from areas which look suspiciously distorted. As in any other facet of life, so in medicine nothing is perfectly straightforward. These distortions are significant only when seen in bowel where inflammation is quiescent; they can be simulated by inflammatory activity and this can give rise to misunderstanding. However, cancer does not develop so quickly, particularly in these circumstances, as to deny the opportunity of another inspection to be undertaken later if the matter is in doubt.

It used to be thought that cancer complicating ulcerative colitis was of a very malignant type; now we know differently. The very considerable interest taken in ulcerative colitis during the years following the war, and the surgical programme which has been pursued, has provided patients whose cases we have been able to study carefully over long periods, in particular following removal of the large intestine in those found to have cancer. From my own practice it has become apparent that the chance of long term survival is possibly better for those developing cancer with ulcerative colitis than it is for a similar group living in the same area who develop large bowel cancer in a previously normal bowel, an observation now being confirmed elsewhere. This difference in favour of ulcerative colitic cancer is intrinsic to the nature of the growth and not due to a better chance of disclosure at an early stage resulting from the newer methods now to hand. This has been revealed by patients in whom cancer was diagnosed and operated upon long before the significance of the mucosal distortion was appreciated and, indeed, before fibre-optic colonoscopes came into being.

5 Trouble beyond the bowel

Inexactitude, seemingly inevitable in psychiatry and the social sciences, sometimes affects other aspects of medical science today; gastroenterology is not exempt. Thus gastric ulcer and duodenal ulcer, two distinct entities, tend to be considered under the one label of 'peptic ulcer' for no better reason than convenience, because they both cause very similar forms of indigestion. So it is with ulcerative colitis and Crohn's disease. Both are now similarly regarded under the one title, 'inflammatory bowel disease', for no better reason than that both are inflammatory conditions involving intestine, both pursue a chronic or repetitive course and both are conditions for which no cause has yet been found. Although Crohn's disease may afflict the colon with appearances resembling the non-specific changes of ulcerative colitis, and although diarrhoea sometimes predominates in Crohn's disease (in only 60 per cent of cases, in effect), while the age at which the two diseases start is similar (Crohn's disease also presents a peak late in life), the two conditions hardly bear a resemblance to one another. Ulcerative colitis is of more ancient lineage; in the last century when micro-organisms were first discovered it became apparent that a dysenteric condition existed of no obvious infectious or parasitic cause; for want of any specific label, ulcerative colitis was what it was called. Crohn's disease was rarely reported before the beginning of this century and was almost unknown until defined by Crohn and his colleagues in 1932, since when its incidence has been alarmingly on the increase, by as much as two- to three-fold in the two decades following 1950; its prevalence is now very similar to that of ulcerative colitis, with a slight preponderance among women.

The sense of convenience which lies behind the modern fashion of lumping the two conditions together can only tend to obscure what clues may lurk in their natural history and in the cellular changes they engender, clues which might shed light on the causation of one or the other or both. Indeed the use of the compendium term distracts attention and awareness from the possibility that such clues of differentiation may exist.

One important difference lies in the lesion itself and the tissue in which it develops. Whereas ulcerative colitis is fundamentally a disease of the mucosa, where the trouble starts with almost immediate ulceration and loss of epithelial surface in the vicinity, the epicentre of Crohn's disease is deeper – in the submucosa. It will be recalled that a thin slip of muscle responsible by its contractions for the unfolding of the mucosa creates a plane, with all the epithelial elements of the crypt glands embedded within the connective tissue stroma on the one side – the luminal side – and on the other an apparent nondescript area containing collections of lymph cells and the nerves to control the muscle wall of the gut. The nondescript area thus delineated by the muscularis mucosa is simply termed the submucosa. It is here that the changes of Crohn's disease begin with an inflammation different in appearance from that seen in ulcerative colitis. It is quieter, it seems to be based on the lymphatic cells set in a ground thickened by the sort of fibrous cells reponsible for scars. Changes do take place at mucosal level but they appear to be ordained by what is developing below and are by no means so widespread as in ulcerative colitis. Indeed the epithelium usually remains intact except here and there – but more of this shortly.

Many diseases have a hallmark, an arrangement and pattern of cells which can be recognised through the microscope as being distinctive; or the causative organism may be observed. Herein lies the *raison d'être* of the pathologist in the care of patients; he can often provide the diagnosis when all else fails and is frequently asked to confirm the diagnosis made by the doctor using samples of tissue, biopsies or specimens removed by the surgeon at operation. The pathologist is not always successful as the final arbiter; his chances of success are greater if such a hallmark can be found and a relevant sample of tissue can be easily obtained.

75

Ulcerative colitis has no hallmark; it presents as a general inflammation. By contrast in Crohn's disease there is what is known as a granuloma, the name given to a grouping of lymphatic and certain other cells easily discernible in localised concentrations. These develop in the submucosa but not in such profusion that they can always be seen in biopsies or specimens; this is particularly true of the large bowel where on occasion it may be impossible to be sure whether a patient with colitis has ulcerative colitis or Crohn's disease. Therein lies yet another reason for the tendency to refer to the two conditions under the one title of 'inflammatory bowel disease', or 'granulomatous disease', a synonym sometimes used with even less justification since in ulcerative colitis inflammatory cells to not congregate in this special way.

Though we have no certain evidence to prove the point, the granuloma of Crohn's disease appears of special import in the development of the condition. It may indicate the starting point of the disturbance which then spreads in the submucosa, for it is at that level that the granulomas are to be seen. The submucosal space then becomes thickened by a reaction which brings in its train the deposition of an inert proteinous material called collagen. Anything going on in the mucosa itself seems of secondary significance; but usually the mucosa is riven here and there by cracks and fissures emanating from the granulomatous submucosa through the mucosa towards the lumen. In this way ulceration develops, but ulceration that is different from what may be seen in ulcerative colitis. There the outer layer of epithelial cells are shed so that the whole surface is lost in affected areas. In Crohn's disease the cracks and fissures present at the mucosal surface as distinctive ulcers and, as might be expected with fissures, those ulcers are not round, nor even roughly so; they are linear, spreading irregularly in the direction of the intestine rather than across it, but intercommunicating with one another leaving intact though swollen mucosa between. This disruptive process begins to proceed in the opposite direction outwards from the submucosa penetrating the circular muscle and beyond; a slow penetration this, not affecting every case and when it does the effect becomes manifest in months or even years, not days.

One feature which distinguishes Crohn's disease from ulcerative colitis is its ubiquity; no part of the alimentary system is immune though in some areas, in particular the gullet and the stomach, it is rare. Moreover the disease may appear outside the gut and show itself in the skin. Ulceration around the anus is perhaps not surprising; but it can develop also at sites remote from the orifices which provide contiguity with the gut, particularly in moist areas such as the flexures of the groin and under the breasts. This is, however, rare.

Dr Crohn and his associates first termed the condition they were describing 'terminal ileitis', appropriately in one respect, for the ileum is the area where the condition most commonly presents itself, either confined there or, as likely as not, spilling over into the large intestine. As befits a chronic disorder the symptoms develop gradually. Ordinarily there is pain at the outset, a pain brought on by a meal and located somewhere across the lower belly; it arises from the inflamed gut itself, and localisation of intestinal pain is imprecise. It may become more precise when the peritoneal lining bounding the abdominal cavity is involved. But in the earlier stage only the gut is affected and that 'reflex' pain accounts for early loss of weight because the patient senses that it is eating which sets it off and so desists before he has become satiated. That may be all – pain and loss of weight, though mild diarrhoea, a loosening of the stool and a slight increase in the number of motions to three or so in the day is usual. At this stage a look at the patient might reveal little wrong to the inexpert eye, though in all probability a parent would observe that their offspring was thin, and might even notice as time went by that the child was not only failing to gain weight but also height.

The faltering nutrition and failure to thrive and grow constitute a concern special to the young patient for if activity of the disease persists without relief puberty may also be delayed. Moreover, if relief is not obtained either naturally or through treatment the teenager may still be undersize when the fusion of the ends of the bones in his limbs takes place, the natural process which brings to an end his growing days. However, this particular problem plays no part in the ailments of an adult.

A glance inside the abdomen at this stage would reveal an area of thickening of the intestine limited in extent, an area where the natural flexibility necessary for its effective function has given way to a rubbery rigidity. The surface would be redder than normal but not notably angry, matching the mild underlying chronic inflammation. This thickening is often detectable; on examining the abdomen the rubbery mass may come to hand; it may be felt for a moment only to slip away as the hand dips deeper to make sure of its presence; it can be tender. This may be the proper moment for confirmation of the diagnosis by x-ray; Crohn's disease in the small intestine is too remote to yield a small biopsy for microscopic examination so that reliance has to be placed upon the circumstantial evidence provided by the features just described together with the x-ray appearances. And that is sufficient to establish the diagnosis since any other cause for these circumstances is unlikely in the extreme.

The x-rays are again obtained by the use of radio-opaque barium sulphate acting as a contrast within the intestinal lumen to reveal the outline of that lumen. But the inconvenience of an enema can be dispensed with; it is a simple matter to swallow the barium made up in a mucilaginous mixture. X-ray photographs are then taken at intervals to match the time likely to be taken for the passage of the barium meal to where the trouble is thought to lie. When it reaches the affected area two features will stand out. The thickening of the submucosa projects both ways so that in addition to the general swelling seen from the peritoneal surface there is also impingement inwards upon the lumen er the full distance that the ileum has become involved, bably a matter of inches, possibly more. So a tube will be probably no more than a quarter of an inch in diameter, if not less, replacing the normal intestinal appearance of a pipe of about half to three quarters of an inch wide feathered at its sides by the enfolding of the mucosa brought about by the muscularis mucosae. The second radiological phenomenon will be observed in the outline: a shallow irregularity will have replaced the slight deep feathering. That irregularity has been formed by ulceration as it takes its wandering course in the area involved between the intact but swollen islands of mucosa, which are thrown up in contrast. As those islands thrust into the lumen they give the impression of a pathway paved with cobblestones.

*

Here, then, is a condition of mild and insidious onset with none of the florid striking features of ulcerative colitis with its dramatic and disabling diarrhoea. Nevertheless 'terminal ileitis' can sometimes be acute. When that happens, as often as not the patient is suspected of having appendicitis and so is admitted to hospital in emergency. For all the appropriate indicators are there – lower abdominal pain starting relatively suddenly, centring upon the right side with tenderness there and vomiting. The discovery when the abdomen is opened that the bowel is the seat of inflammation and not the appendix does not automatically indicate Crohn's disease; there are other causes of acute ileitis, which will be considered later. So the surgeon faced with these circumstances has more than one problem to settle: what the cause of the ileitis may be – and one cause could be yersinial infection mentioned in chapters 1 and 6 – and whether or not to proceed with the operation.

Like ulcerative colitis Crohn's disease follows an unpredictable course. The initial attack may subside of its own accord and not recur for years; when it does the disease may have spread no further. It may, however, crop up again with yet another site of involvement in addition to the one which first appeared in the ileum; indeed a not infrequent development is a further lesion somewhere in the colon. Meanwhile the pathological changes dictate the symptoms. The stricture, for that is virtually what that

79

lengthy narrowing is, takes its toll. The initial pain felt as a result of eating begins to change in character; it becomes sharper, more insistent, more persistent; it has become colic, an indication that the normal progress of food onwards down the alimentary canal is beginning to be held up. This is obstruction of a rather special sort.

In circumstances which more commonly give rise to obstruction, it is brought about by a very localised narrowing; by a growth for example; or by complete obliteration of the lumen by a band or adhesion in the belly acting like a ligature upon the gut. But in Crohn's disease the gauge of the gut is not so reduced as to cause obstruction in this way; it is the distance over which narrowing occurs which gives rise to the trouble. Too much of the intestine becomes inert due to the rigidity of its wall; the ordinary contractions and relaxations which form the peristaltic waves responsible for propelling the contents forward through the gut are stilled. The diameter of the gut is not so reduced as to prevent fluid contents passing through it; but this can only be achieved by the contents being squeezed through by the unaffected gut above, a mechanism which becomes less effective the longer the distance that is diseased. The patient begins to suffer attacks of obstruction usually at times when the disease is more active for then the affected bowel becomes more swollen and inert. When obstruction develops it will probably have to be relieved sooner or later by operation, but not always, for isolated episodes can happen due to some incompletely digested mass getting caught up temporarily within the narrowed segment. This is a circumstance which may not recur.

Meanwhile those cracks in the submucosa proceed outwards as the inflammation progresses; as they approach the peritoneal surface of the affected part penetration of the intestinal wall begins to occur. While this development only rarely leads to perforation, with gut contents flowing freely into the abdominal cavity to induce severe and dangerous peritonitis (this happens in about one to two per cent of cases) it does cause abscesses to form within the peritoneum. These abscesses are contained and surrounded by loops of intestine and whatever else may lie close by, like the urinary bladder. The next stage is the development of a fistula.

A fistula is nothing more nor less than an abnormal communication arising from a hollow organ. That somewhat prosaic description, a hollow organ, covers those parts of the body involved in conducting or containing fluid and any secretory gland. Thus urine may leak onto the skin anywhere from the urinary system: the bladder, the kidney or those little pipes, the ureters, which transport urine from one to the other. The pancreas lies at the back of the abdomen up against the vertebral column where a blow across the upper abdomen can snap it like a twig across the knee – the steering wheel of a car is just the thing to do that. The duct is then severed, the secretions pour out and if luck or surgery prevail these will find their way to the surface where they are likely to digest the skin; but better to digest that than the contents of the abdomen.

There are a variety of causes for abdominal fistula, Crohn's disease being the most potent cause today. For though the disease is still unusual fistula is a common complication when Crohn's disease does occur. Not less than a quarter of all cases sooner or later become affected in this way though not all of them will be afflicted with the distressing problems which arise from faeces or the contents of the small intestine pouring out over the skin.

Intestinal fistula falls into two main categories, particularly in Crohn's disease, because the inflammatory process which presages the fistula is as likely to cause adherence of the affected gut to a neighbouring organ inside the abdomen as to the abdominal wall. The first leads to an internal fistula, the second to an external one, with quite different consequences. In some circumstances the effects of an internal fistula are trivial, as when the ileum opens into the large intestine nearby. The terminal ileum lies in close juxtaposition alongside that part of the large intestine, the caecum and ascending colon, into which it normally discharges its contents. An additional opening there, though abnormal, will make little difference. Quite often an ileal fistula spreads further afield to a more distant area, the sigmoid colon. Although this is anatomically speaking on the other side of the abdomen and in terms of the gut is far removed, the two structures lie in close proximity as they hang down side by side into the pelvis. So a sizeable length of gut is circumvented but the fistula is seldom of significance because it rarely creates an effective shunt. But this incursion from the ileum does often set off a new focus of activity in the colon. Perhaps the involvement of caecum and ascending colon so often seen in continuity with ileitis is partly contributed to in the same way, by the short fistulas emanating from the original site of trouble in the ileum.

It would be a mistake to dismiss as innocuous all internal fistulas involving only the gut; it depends upon the extent to which intestinal contents are shunted along the fortuitous channel and away from parts of the gut with important functions to perform. This seldom happens in Crohn's disease because the fistulous track is usually too narrow to allow much of the viscid contents to pass through even from the small bowel. Thus it is that a fistula between ileum and sigmoid, though it bypasses much of the colon, seldom leads to diarrhoea on that account, a circumstance to be expected when so considerable an area responsible for the absorption of water has been excluded. A wider channel would cause or aggravate diarrhoea; in addition scarring in the gut beyond the upper end of a fistula could cause a hold up with a tendency to divert the intestinal contents down the wrong way.

More serious is a 'high' fistula, by which is meant a track connected to the upper intestine. This can materialise as far up as the duodenum; which may seem strange when the disease is active at a site as distant as the ileum. The two areas are not normally in anatomical relationship to one another; indeed they are separated by a matter of inches. But they become much closer as disease in the ascending colon progresses, for this does lie in close proximity to the duodenum. As it becomes shortened by scarring, so the conglomerate mass of thickened infected tissue incorporating ileum and ascending colon comes to lie close enough for a connection to form between ileum and colon and the duodenum. A situation now develops which can have serious effects: diarrhoea becomes marked and contains fat. The patient loses weight noticeably, an outward and visible sign that important digestive and absorptive functions are impaired.

This is not due to the shunting of duodenal contents directly into the colon; another mechanism is at work. Colonic bacteria have gained access to the normally sterile reaches of the upper small intestine; this contamination not only causes fat to be broken down to fatty acids which the body cannot handle so that fat is excreted instead of being absorbed, but also damages the sensitive mucosa so that it loses its luxuriance, becomes flattened and attenuated, and much digestive and absorptive capacity is lost. No longer can protein molecules be cut up neatly into their constituent amino-acids and fully utilised; nitrogenous material – the possession of nitrogen atoms distinguishes protein from fat and carbohydrate – begins to appear in quantity in the stool; normally one gram of nitrogen is lost in the stool each day, this representing no more than the protein shed from the walls of the gut when mucosal cells inevitably die, and that contained in the bodies of bacteria lost in the faecal draught. When protein is forfeited in quantity the patient begins to lose weight rapidly.

This is not the only means whereby internal fistula can be more than a nuisance. The ileo-sigmoid fistula is in close proximity to the bladder. How easy for that organ to become incorporated in the phlegmonous mass created by the nearby inflammation. The first indication of involvement will be a tetchiness of the bladder: in addition to diarrhoea a desire to pass urine more often, sometimes incurring pain: demands occurring at night with consequent loss of sleep, in all probability already disturbed by diarrhoea. All gets worse as the fistula breaks through to discharge into the bladder itself. Theoretically urine could pass into the colon when the bladder is full and cannot be emptied, for the desire to pass water is occasioned by rhythmic contractions of the bladder wall of ever increasing intensity. Maybe this does happen; if so, only a little urine escapes and it passes unobserved in the stool. The trouble arises in the opposite direction; intestinal gas is pushed from colon to bladder so that little puffs of wind are noticed to the surprise of the victim as he passes water. Women, for reasons which must be obvious, are less likely to notice this or a later development – what appears to be and is faeces in the urine.

In these several ways the internal fistula can make itself more than felt. Clearly an abscess which evolves towards the abdominal wall and breaks out onto the surface to open up a connection between the bowel lumen and the skin can be a greater source of disability. Again there is a saving grace; not every external fistula causes gut contents to escape, and those that do often do so intermittently. Moreover the harmful effects of an active external fistula vary according to its level – the higher the worse.

Because the ileum provides the commonest site in which the disease embeds itself, lesions in this area have been taken as the examples of what may happen generally. But it may break out anywhere between mouth and anus. In about twenty per cent of cases it is the jejunum which is involved; an external fistula from this area will be more likely to leak because jejunal contents are fluid, and as they ooze out upon the skin the effect will be similar to a pancreatic fistula. The digestive enzymes will excoriate the skin, while the persistent moisture macerates it. Although it is more difficult to cure the ulceration of the skin which results than prevent it, this can be done by the judicious use of modern adhesive materials which are protective to the skin and enable a thin plastic bag to be attached over the opening to collect the fluid and drain it away from the susceptible skin. The bags, which are designed for the management and control of surgical stomas (see chapter 7), are frequently used for external fistulas communicating with the colon not so much because the faecal effluent is enough to require a receptacle of this nature but as a dressing which prevents underclothes becoming soiled

84

and also keeps odour under control. The passage of faeces from fistulas of the colon and ileum tends to be intermittent, pus alternating with it. The eruptions cease for a few days at a time, then longer, events which begin to herald closure by natural remission.

*

There are many aspects to Crohn's disease: it is not just another form of dysentery like ulcerative colitis. The symptoms which announce its presence may not at first reveal their cause. Although unusual, what may first draw attention to the condition is fever, without any clear indication of how this has come about because of a dearth of symptoms to point to the gut as being the site of the trouble. Several other conditions can declare themselves in this way, typhoid and tuberculosis amongst them.

Crohn's disease can start in so many different ways. Sometimes the onset is insidious so that the patient but gradually becomes aware that something is amiss; anaemia gradually bringing in its train a sense of tiredness and no more than that at first, with shortness of breath on exertion to follow later. Added to that may be the weakness and inertia of prolonged interference with digestive absorption, though in that circumstance these vague symptoms are likely to be compounded by diarrhoea due to the fatty stools.

Who would expect a disease of the intestine to start with a limp? Though unusual, it is a fair example of the way in which an intestinal disorder can affect other systems. The limp comes about when an area of ileitis lies close by a muscle at the back of the abdomen acting upon the right leg to bring about certain movements of the right hip. The nearby inflammation limits the freedom of this muscle preventing the hip from being straightened completely; any attempt to do so brings on pain.

By spreading in this direction the disease can invade other structures, notably the right kidney and its ureter where that tube passes over the selfsame muscle towards the bladder. Urinary symptoms then occur, either from infection of the kidney, so that the individual suffers the common symptoms of that complaint, frequently passing water and feeling pain on doing so; or the ureter becomes caught up in the chronic inflammation of the intestine and is strangled by it to the extent that the flow of urine from the kidney is blocked. Again there is pain, but this time from the kidney, pain that is felt in the loin.

These manifestations are in a sense secondary phenomena, brought about by juxtaposition. The possibility that Crohn's disease is the cause of symptoms may be overlooked because of the area in which it is located. Sometimes, though rarely, the duodenum is the focus, when the ensuing symptoms simulate the common duodenal ulcer in more ways than one; and the same goes for an even rarer site of involvement – the stomach. Because of the very rarity of the disease in these situations the possibility may not be borne in mind, though the abnormalities demontrated in the duodenum by x-rays or direct vision through a gastroscope should be sufficiently unusual to implant the idea.

A description of the numerous and variable manifestations of this ubiquitous disease would be overwhelming. Suffice it to say that because Crohn's disease does also attack the colon in a manner not unlike ulcerative colitis, though in a less florid way, there is a coincidence between the two as regards symptoms and acute complications. Disintegration of the colonic wall with dilatation, perforation releasing gut contents into the peritoneal cavity, and haemorrhage – all these emergencies of ulcerative colitis may also bedevil Crohn's disease. Furthermore haemorrhage can happen in the small intestine, which can also become perforated by the same penetrative process that leads to fistula. Cancer is also an increased risk in both small and large intestine in those who have suffered Crohn's disease for many years, and probably for the same reason: namely, that persistent inflammation causes a faster rate of 'turnover' of epithelial cells in the mucosa. As more cells are needed to replace those being lost they begin to distort. Subsequent generations of cells carry the stigma of this distortion; so premalignant changes take place from which new lines of cancer cells are born, new malignant clones.

All the while the chances of complications involving anatomically remote tissues and organs like the skin, eyes, joints and the liver may develop as in ulcerative colitis.

*

There is a tendency to another sort of fistula – at the anus; this is as common as the abdominal fistula, indeed more so. All those in whom the rectum is affected will at some time in the course of their disease have trouble at the anus, either in the form of ulceration or fistulation. The further the site of the intestinal lesion from the anus the lower the probability of trouble developing there; nevertheless a quarter of those with ileitis will suffer anal trouble of one sort or another.

Anal fistula starts just inside the back passage. Slowly, over months, it runs into the surrounding tissue in a somewhat haphazard fashion, so that an opening appears on the surface anywhere in the vicinity; often more than one opening is produced. It has a habit of moving towards the vagina or the base of the scrotum. Whether or not those areas are involved, the outcome is a discharge of pus and sometimes faeces in that region. With it goes soreness, while from time to time small abscesses break down to reveal yet other openings into the fistulous system.

These troubles cause much distress over and above any actual discomfort, which is fortunately rather less than might be expected; but this is small mitigation for the embarrassment, the sense of shame and of stigma which any disturbance in the anal and vaginal areas must cause. The social and psychological problems are worse for a woman; her relationships with men or within marriage may be threatened or she is likely to fear that they may be. Apart from the obvious discouragement to love-making, a discharge in the area between the legs (the perineum) must cause the situation to be complicated by pain on intercourse (dyspareunia) when the fistula runs close to the vagina. In addition pressure upon a tender section of gut through the abdominal wall, or through the vagina on penetration of the penis, is another cause of dyspareunia. The problem is more than compounded by the development of an outright opening into the vagina brought about when a recto-vaginal fistula occurs.

There are other ways in which Crohn's disease brings social stress in its train; it is not difficult to imagine the strains within a family imposed by the persistent illness of a wife and mother, and by her inability to cope with the misunderstandings arising therefrom because of her weariness and inertia due to anaemia, loss of energy and malaise. Add to that the crippling effect of diarrhoea when it occurs. All these disabilities call for a degree of understanding and compassion from her partner which is unlikely to be forthcoming where love no longer exists to fortify the partnership; where it does, the problems are shared and the ties of the partnership become stronger – one redeeming feature in a daunting situation.

The single woman no less than a man is faced with the problem of earning. The earner may be able to continue at work if the job is sedentary though getting to work can be difficult, for there is no medical contraindication on physical grounds to continuing to work. Sometimes depression supervenes, though not so very often, and saps the will to work. The plight of the individual with ulcerative colitis is worse, for during an attack diarrhoea predominates and is likely to do so to an extent which must rob her of the capacity to work. Only if the condition is mild can the patient continue at work.

Children inflicted with either disease have greater problems. Diarrhoea is a symptom which may subject the sufferer to ridicule from uncomprehending school fellows who regard with derision repeated requests to leave the classroom to go to the toilet. There is the added strain of maintaining continence; the occasional inevitable 'accident' occurs. Time is taken off from school which may appear less serious than for an adult who has to stay away from work; the occasional absence inevitable in childhood is of little consequence but when repeated or prolonged it becomes a matter of concern because it puts the child's future at hazard. Crucial examinations may be missed, or standards obtained below the individual's capacity, thus jeopardising university entry. While the adult loses earnings the child forfeits future earning capacity.

Ulcerative colitis and Crohn's disease resemble one another in the incapacities they inflict; in this respect the compendium 'inflammatory bowel disease' is justified.

---

6 Cancer and other matters

There is a finite limit to the number of cells required by any organ, numerous though they may normally be. Thus the liver stops growing at a size commensurate with the requirements and demands of the corporate whole it serves. The liver is easily damaged by drugs, alcohol and other poisonous substances, to say nothing of the viruses which are now so commonly and easily passed from man to man to cause hepatitis. In the illness which follows, liver cells are destroyed and lost, but once the disorder is overcome their replacement is achieved by those cells which have weathered the storm replicating themselves until the gap, so to speak, has been filled. When that has been achieved the process ceases and all the cells, both new and old, return to normal duties. This switch-on switch-off process is at the command of the cell nucleus where the information required to activate it is inscribed in the DNA of the nucleus. A graze of the skin or a burn is healed by the same process. Indeed with few exceptions self-replication is part of the normal activity of cells in any tissue or organ in order to replace those lost naturally by wear and tear, and also to expand to meet increased demand, as muscles have to do in response to continued activity.

But things can go wrong; the nucleus of a cell can lose control through lapse of its appreciation of the proper place in the order of things of the cell it controls. No longer does the presence of its neighbours stop the cell going too far, through an indefinable sense of juxtaposition. A new line of cells is formed which go on reproducing themselves unchecked, and a malignant line comes into being. Meanwhile the malignant identity becomes stamped upon these cells, visible as a change in shape and increased density of the nucleus. It becomes all too apparent that the nucleus is the flaw in the distortion of these rogue cells. Invasion of the parent tissue begins, to be followed by progress into the organ of which the tissue forms a part, and as time passes, beyond into the surrounding structures. The more malignant the cancer, the more invasive it is and the more obvious does the nuclear material become, to the exclusion of the rest of the cell. In this way cells of a malignant growth lose their ordinary function.

It is a fact of life that epithelial cells are more susceptible to malignant change than connective tissue, which comprises artery, nerve, muscle and bone. This is understandable in epithelial tissue of the skin, which is particularly subject to all forms of radiation from the sun and, in addition, a variety of chemical abuses, any of which may set the nuclear material off on the wrong track: probably by interference at the vulnerable moment when the nuclear material lines up in chromosomes in order to split to provide two sets for cell division. The reason for cancer developing in epithelium in the more sheltered reaches of the intestine is less obvious, though there is a clue: malignancy is rare in the small intestine but common in the large where the epithelial cells are subject to constant bacterial and viral damage absent from normal small bowel.

Cancer of the large bowel is common; so it plays an inevitable role in the story of the flux in addition to the diagnostic confusion that can occur between it and the chronic inflammatory diseases, and the increased malignant potential latent in them. It is more a disease of western society; the food we take may be playing a part, fat in particular being indicted in a rather indirect way which links diet and the bacterial flora of the gut.

Bile, which is the product of the breakdown of haemoglobin by the liver, is put to good use when it is excreted into the gut. Some of the chemical salts of bile assist vitamin absorption, others fat absorption by emulsification of fatty acids. Bile salts should be absorbed by the time they reach the end of the small bowel, to return to a pool in the liver for reuse while the pigments pass on to be excreted with the stool, giving faeces their characteristic colour. If too much fat is eaten, the component fatty acids get carried further, beyond the ileo-caecal valve and into the large bowel in conjunction with bile acids which have no business there. Colonic bacteria fall upon the bile acids degrading them into substances noxious to the cells of the colon. In the fullness of time some of these epithelial cells begin to change, possibly because of increased turnover due to replacement of cells damaged by the degraded bile. Little wart-like excrescences, polyps so-called, begin to make their appearance on the luminal surface of the colon, at first little more than a mound of cells somewhat altered in shape but with no invasive tendency. That comes later. It is all very similar to the reaction in the skin of an individual sensitive to light or overexposed to it, when ultimately the surface cells begin to heap up into something akin to a wart, termed hyperkeratosis, which similarly represents the preinvasive stage of cancer.

Three things happen as large bowel malignancy develops. It makes its presence felt either in the form of a tumour or an ulcer or a stricture. All are conducive to a variety of symptoms from obstructive colic to the looseness of diarrhoea and the exhaustion associated with the anaemia of constant slow blood loss. Any resemblance between large bowel cancer and ulcerative colitis is remote, however, for though both give rise to anaemia the pattern of diarrhoea is different in each condition with more urgency and frequency in the ulcerative colitis. The symptomatic picture presented by Crohn's disease may overlap that of malignancy here and there but not so closely as to mislead the diagnostician into confusing the two, particularly by the time he has undertaken his clinical examination.

*

Simulations can be the bugbear of the diagnostician. Consider ileocaecal tuberculosis, the chronic infection from which regional ileitis was plucked by Dr Crohn. There is no dissimilarity in symptoms; the x-ray resemblance between the two is usually identical; in both it may be possible to feel the affected area through the abdominal wall. All of which is hardly surprising since the microscopic picture of the two diseases, though not identical, is so alike. There was a time here in the UK when abdominal tuberculosis seemed a thing of the past, but it made its comeback with the very considerable immigration from the Asian continent. Now it is necessary to exclude tuberculosis as a cause of ileitis before making the diagnosis of Crohn's disease in an Indian or a Pakistani. How important it is to do so. Tuberculosis can be cured with the appropriate antibiotics while we are powerless to do more than ease the symptoms of a patient with Crohn's disease. To achieve the diagnosis an operation to open the abdomen may be necessary so that a direct view of the abnormal bowel can be obtained with, possibly, a snippet of affected tissue for microscopic study and confirmation of the diagnosis, although tuberculosis can usually be identified by what presents itself to the naked eye.

Just as tuberculosis was found to be not the sole cause of ileitis we have now become aware that acute ileitis is not the sole prerogative of Crohn's disease, as used to be thought. It takes time for such matters to come to light; the natural history of a chronic disease can only be fully observed over a life time. It could be said that a life time has now passed since Crohn's disease was described in 1932, certainly a professional life time, and although Dalziel's description of the chronic interstitial enteritis defined a chronic disease, Crohn and his colleagues described four different types, one of which was an acute form indistinguishable from acute appendicitis and defying diagnosis until acute ileitis was disclosed at operation. So the concept that acute ileitis was *ipso facto* Crohn's disease became imbued in medical minds until time showed that many of these acute cases, possibly up to 80 per cent, cleared up without further ado.

Time also showed Crohn's disease to be a recurrent illness, thus disestablishing that 80 per cent. *Yersinia enterocolitica* (chapter 1) began to make itself felt in Scandinavia in the 1960s as a cause of enteritis and so of diarrhoea; its territory began to spread to other countries where it had either not been seen before or had not been identified, for it is not the easiest species to identify when it causes trouble. It was then realised that yersinia was responsible for at least some of those cases of acute ileitis. So it has become a matter of importance to establish the involvement of this organism in any individual with this disorder for it can be treated with an antibiotic if it fails to subside of its own accord. Moreover it does not recur; nor have we any evidence that the ileitis it causes, which looks so like Crohn's disease in appearance, extent and site in the small intestine, predisposes to Crohn's disease later.

No doubt until fairly recent times we were mistaking ischaemic for ulcerative colitis, for the condition had remained unrecognised. Ischaemia is a medical code word for what happens when the blood supply becomes deficient. It will be familiar to many in ischaemic heart disease, a title which conjures up the unpleasantness of angina and may include catastrophic episodes such as coronary thrombosis; all this when the blood supply through the arteries to the heart (the coronary arteries) is reduced through their narrowing by arteriosclerosis or actual occlusion by clotting. The elderly, and younger people who smoke heavily, can suffer gangrene of a leg due to the same trouble elsewhere in the arterial system – another example of ischaemia. Deprivation of blood supply so that additional demands for oxygen and nutrients made by increasing activity of an organ or tissue cannot be met, may affect many a vital organ.

The intestines are not exempt though in normal circumstances they are richly endowed as regards blood supply; they need to be with all that absorption going on. But even there, important vessels supplying large areas of gut may become narrowed or even shut off as they branch away from the main supply. Then the affected area has to rely upon blood being brought in from the adjacent regions of bowel by other vessels which may be defective too, a situation which can lead to all-out gangrene or, if limited in effect, to a localised stricture. These manifestations of intestinal ischaemia have been recognised for what they are, for many years: the limited effect may ultimately come to resemble Crohn's disease; otherwise they are not our concern in the story of the flux. What is new, or relatively so, is the recognition that ischaemia of the bowel can present in another and more insidious way.

Gangrene, whether complete or incomplete, is the result of the whole thickness of the bowel wall dying from the effect of blood deprivation. Now we know that under certain circumstances the mucosa alone may die and that this can happen particularly in circumstances when the blood pressure falls and remains low for long enough to jeopardise the flow through that system of communicating vessels in the submucosa from which the supply passes inwards to the mucosa itself. It does not do for the mucosa of the colon to remain unprotected for too long in this way; its resistance to attack from the organisms in the lumen is weakened. Parts of the mucosa then die leaving the colon denuded here and there or over wider areas. Bloody diarrhoea marks the moment when those defective patches of mucosa slough away, to continue in a manner resembling ulcerative colitis so closely as to be indistinguishable except by x-rays; a barium enema, done at an early stage may display a shape to those ulcers and their distribution in the bowel unlike that seen in ulcerative colitis. The coup which lowers the pressure may be a sudden illness; it may come from prolonged operations when blood loss is imperfectly controlled, as I have seen following hip replacement and heart operations.

There is a strange, equivocal but common condition seen all too often in gastrointestinal clinics throughout the world, strange because it presents no obvious abnormality despite the patient's bowel complaints, and equivocal because of the inconsistency of those complaints. At one moment the patient has diarrhoea, at the next constipation;

wind and colic may compound either. Diarrhoea when it occurs is mild, no more than some increase in the number of bowel actions daily. Patients often complain that they pass fluid stools but the faecal content is formed and the cause is an unusual abundance of intestinal mucus. It used to pass under the name 'spastic colon', but this has given way in recent times to 'the irritable bowel syndrome' in order to include a wider sphere of involvement than the large bowel alone. We are ordinarily unaware of the activity of our gut. The abnormality of the irritable bowel syndrome bringing on the symptoms of wind and colic may be the consciousness of normal bowel activity.

The trouble about the irritable bowel syndrome is that it is a disorder of little consequence but considerable disturbance; since those who suffer, fear not unreasonably that something substantial, something organic, must be amiss. Their symptoms lead to investigation – endoscopy and x-rays – only to reveal nothing wrong. What can the doctors be missing? That is the next thought: a thought, which arouses a sense of insecurity, of failure of confidence, giving rise to a twinge of fear too easily transmitted into a suspicion that something sinister is lurking unrevealed: 'it must be cancer'. In truth it is nothing of the sort, but doubt engenders reluctance to accept reassurance so that the real symptoms worsen without organic cause. It is difficult for these patients to appreciate that there is nothing wrong or that they are not being told, in effect, that their troubles are imaginary. That is why the tendency today is to avoid investigation if possible; it is only required when the complaints raise a real possibility that something else may be amiss (Crohn's disease can be one possibility). The nuisance value of the irritable bowel syndrome lies less in the discomfort it causes than the concern. The best treatment lies with the doctor who is prepared to listen, who is able to recognise the condition from the story, who has the strength of mind to avoid recourse to investigation and, last but by no means least, who will spend as much time as is needed to explain the situation. It is remarkable how the symptoms ease to tolerable proportions, if not totally, when suspicion and fear are properly allayed.

The earlier title, spastic colon, had been ascribed to the condition on a symptomatic basis in the absence of anything substantial that could be found wrong in any other way. It had to be changed because it led to confusion when spasm of the colon could be demonstrated by x-rays, in particular as part of the chain of events leading to diverticulitis, a condition which has been known to be simulated by Crohn's disease. It most commonly affects the colon, particularly the sigmoid area where the changes seen on barium enema sometimes bear a close resemblance.

Diverticulitis is a misleading designation since the inflammation indicated by this appellation is but secondary to mechanical changes of a truly spastic nature, causing small out-pouches to protrude from the bowel wall. These diverticula are brought about by mucosa being pushed outwards alongside the arteries and veins where they penetrate the muscle wall of the colon; here are areas of potential weakness which give way when localised spasms of the circular muscle bite deep into the lumen to cause intervening circumscribed areas of high pressure. From time to time the neck of a diverticulum becomes blocked so that it no longer has free access to get rid of its secretions back into the colonic channel. That is when infection can occur and diverticular disorder becomes diverticulitis.

But here is one disorder which is on the wane. In palaeographic terms it has not been with us for long. It was of our own making when sugar was made sweeter by refinement and bread whiter, and supposedly more palatable. Milling with iron rollers spread from Hungary to replace stone rolling in the late nineteenth century so that the bran of the wheat husk could then be removed from the middlings and semolinas of the kernel before the flour was formed. Through these and other eliminations of fibre from western diets we have become heirs to numerous common conditions today, diverticular disorder being one, a cause of mucus diarrhoea which should not be a source of trouble for much longer.

PART TWO

The treatment of chronic diarrhoea

7 Ulcerative colitis

Where the cause of a disease is known, treatment may present a problem; when it is unknown and the condition is chronic with a tendency to relapse we can do little more than grope in the dark and clutch at straws. Most diarrhoea is epidemic, a bacterial infection caught through contaminated food or water, or a viral intrusion acquired from the next man. These are seldom fatal; in many cases it matters little whether a specific remedy, the antibiotic appropriate to the organism, is taken or not since the condition is self-limiting. Indeed there is much to be said for avoiding antibiotics if possible since their administration tends to deny the development of natural immunity and also disturbs the bacterial population in the gut allowing other, less congenial organisms to take over vacant possession. This is the policy in dealing with traveller's diarrhoea, though if the drugs which calm the gut and so diminish both discomfort and diarrhoea are ineffective, more specific measures may be called for to cut short the inconvenience, discomfort and disability. Isolation is sometimes necessary to stop the spread of an epidemic, particularly in institutions with a 'captive' population, or in an outbreak of an illness of more serious import like typhoid when antibiotic treatment is likely to be used at the outset – at the moment the diagnosis is made or suspected. This underlines the importance of establishing or eliminating an infective cause as soon as possible.

Cholera provides one example of a dangerous disease where it may be politic not to use an antibiotic since the vibrio readily develops resistance and thus persistance. It can be a serious matter if antibiotic-resistant bacteria of the cholera family are encouraged to develop in a community during an epidemic. The appropriate drug, tetracycline, will halve the amount of fluid lost by a patient through diarrhoea by the simple process of reducing the number of viable vibrios. But the immune processes we are endowed with will actually eliminate them, given time, provided fluid is given by vein or mouth in volume sufficient to match the loss and so keep the patient alive while the body gathers the appropriate immunological strength.

So the first essential step is to make a diagnosis; this is not always easy and sometimes is only possible by inference. Circumstances may delay, deny or even prevent the necessary samples of stool being examined to establish the cause in a case of dysentery or food poisoning. When the cause is a virus, identification presents a greater problem. Bacteria grow quickly and with relative ease in or on media laced with the appropriate sugar, spice and all things nice for the bacterium. Not so with viruses, which enjoy the living cell and little else, so that they have to be grown on cell cultures. This is not easy and takes a considerable time, so long in fact that the victim has recovered by the time the organism is identified. In terms of the patient's care this matters little since the disturbance caused by viral diarrhoea seldom lasts longer than a day or two and has no serious consequences. The only danger lies in the temptation for the doctor to prescribe an antibiotic, a useless gesture since none has yet been found to deal with a virus.

By comparison how negative must our attitude inevitably be to ulcerative colitis or Crohn's disease. We just do not know where to begin or which way to turn other than using remedies known to ease diarrhoea by their tendency to 'bind' the bowels, such as the opiates or the more innocuous chalk, or codeine, particularly as these diseases are recurrent and will persist on and off throughout life. That could be stated the other way round, placing the emphasis more upon remission than relapse, by accentuating the trouble-free periods, which can last a long time, even up to years. This attitude concentrates the therapeutic approach more upon the need to bring about a remission and the easement of symptoms, and then upon how to keep a patient in remission. By trial and error over many years, two drugs have been found to be useful in this respect for ulcerative colitis.

100

It was in the 1930s that the antibiotic era started with the introduction of the sulphonamide group of drugs, Prontosil being the first. Overnight almost, streptococcal infections were robbed of their terror; today they hardly ever come to the fore except in some cases of sore throat. As with penicillin, which was to appear in the next decade, numerous analogues of sulphonamide were developed and tested against other organisms. The sulphonamide family grew rapidly. In 1941 a Swedish physician Dr Nanna Swartz, began to take an interest in the sulphonamides and found one, salazopyrine (officially known as sulphasalazine) which brought about a good response in ulcerative colitis, more particularly the milder cases and those with disease limited to only a part of the large bowel. At the time it was thought that sulphasalazine was ridding the bowel of a noxious but unidentified bacterium or, maybe, reducing the number of bowel organisms generally and so reducing the contamination of the ulcers in the mucosa, so that during a respite they could heal. For there were still lingering thoughts that ulcerative colitis could be a form of dysentery. Dr Bargen of the Mayo Clinic – the man who sat next to Dr Crohn in New Orleans – had described a special bacterium in the stool of ulcerative colitis patients not ordinarily to be found in the normal bowel. Although Bargen's bacillus was soon ruled out the thought remained that the cause was infective. It was on that premise that sulphasalazine was tried and found to be helpful; symptoms were eased and the inflammation of the mucosa in the rectum was seen to subside and often entirely disappear.

Forty years have elapsed and the means whereby sulphasalazine achieves its effect are still imperfectly understood though one thing we do know; it is not by any bactericidal activity. It now seems likely that it exercises some control over the inflammatory response associated with the immune mechanisms within the mucosa. Maybe that is why its most useful function is in prolonging a remission; once an attack of ulcerative colitis has been brought under control sulphasalazine is used to keep it under control – maintenance therapy, in professional jargon.

There is a snag, one which after so long has only been discovered, virtually by chance, in the last five years due to an observation made by a patient and his doctors pursuing it. For two years or more he had been receiving sulphasalazine to prevent further recurrence. At the same time it was of some concern to him that his wife was not conceiving. Since his colitis was remaining quiescent the drug was withdrawn. Shortly afterwards his wife became pregnant. This important observation led to the examination of spermatic fluid of patients receiving this drug; the sperm count was reduced, and distorted forms of spermatozoa were present indicating interference with their development. This effect, however, is not permanent; within a month or more of stopping the drug all goes back to normal. So maintenance therapy now has to be fitted in with planning a family. What has not yet been pursued is the possibility that here is a male oral contraceptive in the making.

A decade passed before a whole new area of therapy opened up with the introduction of corticosteroids – substances developed in the adrenal gland. Never before had we had at our disposal drugs known to diminish inflammation. It was not long before they were being used for ulcerative colitis. Today an acute episode is treated with those steroids known as prednisone and prednisolone, with reasonable expectation that the attack will subside; thereafter the steroids cease to be taken and are replaced by sulphasalazine in the hope that the remission gained by the steroids will thus be maintained. Milder manifestations of the disease may respond to the sulpha drug given alone from the outset.

There are circumstances when medical treatment will not suffice, either because the patient fails to respond to the drugs, or gets worse, or remission cannot be maintained so that relapses develop ever more frequently. The reasons why the situation can run out of medical control are numerous. A complication like arthritis of the knee or spine may develop and will only be corrected by removal of the large intestine; after ten to fifteen years cancer becomes an in-

creasing hazard and that calls for elimination of the offending organ. There can be no hard and fast rules or guidelines
to surgery, which is the next stage. Each patient is an
individual presenting different problems arising from the
one disease. Social problems vary: loss of time from education is more disastrous than time off work later in life.
Frequent episodes of diarrhoea are less tolerable in the
young; they may constitute a reason for contemplating
operation at an earlier stage than in an adult.

*

There is only one logical operation for ulcerative colitis
which has been proved fully effective – removal of the large
bowel *in toto*. There have been others no less logical
perhaps, certainly less absolute, but ineffective in the
event. Removal in part, which would seem reasonable
when only a segment of the large intestine is diseased, is
doomed to failure because the disorder ultimately recurs in
what colon remains with distressing inevitability. It was a
reasonable thought that diversion of intestinal contents
away from the ulcerated bowel, through a special opening
on the surface of the abdomen made for the purpose from
the small intestine, would cause a respite from faecal contamination of the ulcers so that they might heal. In the
event they did not; severe general effects were in part
mitigated thereby but seldom for long. When, happily, a
prolonged remission did follow, attempts to restore normality by getting rid of the artificial opening were always
defeated by relapse.

The next move was to take advantage of such an opening
to pour salves and medicaments through it in the hope that
these would promote healing. The concept of irrigation of
the bowel in this way was not new, it had been put into
practice at the beginning of the century by an American
surgeon who in 1902 had the ingenious idea of using the
appendix for the purpose. The appendix is a tube considerably narrower than the small intestine, but it has a channel
big enough to allow a catheter to be passed through it; so
why not bring this to the surface? Though the organ is very
variable in length it is usually long enough for this to be

done. For the next forty years this operation, appendicostomy, persisted with no evidence that the solutions and substances varying from sodium bicarbonate to cod-liver oil (without the malt!) poured through appendices the world over had any effect whatsoever. For those were still the days of the art of surgery rather than of critical assessment – which is happily now beginning to prevail.

The artificial opening for faecal deflection, an ileostomy, was achieved by the simple procedure of bringing the last part of the ileum out onto the surface in a loop into which the opening was made. This proved to be a disaster in itself for one reason: the contents of the small bowel are fluid; it was impossible to contain or in any way control these excretions. Leakage occurred constantly beyond voluminous dressings placed around the ileostomy to prevent this, so that the skin around the stoma ulcerated beneath what in effect became a faecal poultice.So ileostomy was reserved as a life-saving measure, which in the event it seldom proved to be. Surgery had little more to offer than medicine – and at that time sulphasalazine was yet to be invented. Why were these operations even considered? *Faute-de-mieux*, in hope more than in expectation, and because an operation does encourage all concerned with the feeling that something is being done, for it is difficult simply to stand by in masterly inactivity. Then in 1944 one patient changed all that, a young chemistry student named Koenig.

*

For centuries one artificial bowel opening, colostomy, had dominated the medical scene to the exclusion of all others, if only because other stomas were rarely needed or rarely established because of the difficulty of controlling them: ileostomy being an obvious case in point and nephrostomy – a hole made into the kidney to drain away urine – another, even more unmanageable (since a nephrostomy has to be sited inaccessibly in the back). Accounts of colostomy exist which go back to the eighteenth century and no doubt openings into the large bowel were made long before that in order to relieve large bowel obstruction (almost always due to cancer) when all other remedies had failed. Those other remedies were numerous and drastic; physicians from the beginning of time have wielded effective purgatives. Salts, senna, aloes, colocynth, jalap, scammony, gamboge, elaterium and calomel were all tried out on a 64 year old widow of Bath – also quicksilver, advantage being taken of the weight of the mercury with the intent of breaking through the obstruction.

Even this failed but not before the widow had received enough mercury to cause her teeth to fall out – a sign of mercury poisoning. The physicians had met their Waterloo (appropriately, for it was shortly after 1815) so a Mr Pringle was called in to operate. He made a colostomy on the left side, doubtless bringing out a loop of colon there, with the triumphant words: 'It was a ticklish business and required throughout a very nice steerage.'

The widow was the first English patient known to have survived a colostomy. Pringle may even have got his mercury back, an important point in those days for it must have been expensive. In 1776 a French patient had been stood on his head in an attempt to recover two pounds of quicksilver he had had to swallow but it was lost for ever, probably because Monsieur Pillore, surgeon of Rouen, made the colostomy on the right side, too far above the site of obstruction. Probably for the same reason the patient died a month after operation – the first recorded instance of the institution of a large bowel stoma.

The difficulties of the operation must have been considerable, for there were no anaesthetics. But there was no particular difficulty about the management of a large bowel stoma especially if placed on the left side of the abdomen. Large bowel contents are solid or semisolid by the time they reach the left colon, containable therefore in dressings placed over a colostomy though this is hardly required in most cases. Although there is no way in which the muscles of the abdominal wall can be reconstructed around a colostomy so as to create a new valve to emulate the anus, simply because this requires a sensory component we cannot provide, nevertheless the large bowel retains a rhythmicity of action which allows the bowels to open fairly predictably once or twice a day after breakfast or a morning cup of tea, and sometimes a later meal. Indeed bowel actions can be anticipated to some extent with greater certainty than by those who retain normal rectal function, since the colostomy patient is less likely to become costive, and if he does he can be trained to undertake the more tedious performance of a daily bowel washout. So a colostomy needs only a light cover; dressings to contain a bowel motion are hardly needed.

Back in 1824 a book-keeper in Blackburn who had had a colostomy brought out in the left groin to relieve obstruction due to cancer of the rectum was provided with a truss by his surgeon Martland to hold a small tin box over the stoma, but the patient found a small sponge held in place by a bandage better. To all intents and purposes that is where matters have remained, no special appliance having been designed for colostomy other than a large corset to fix a shallow cup over the stoma – a substitute for the tin box. None of this made the management of an ileostomy a practicality until the situation was changed by Koenig.

For many years a Chicago surgeon, Strauss, had taken an interest in ulcerative colitis; indeed twenty years earlier he had described how in three patients he had removed the whole colon at one operation (it was usual in those days when surgery was a desultory event in the treatment of ulcerative colitis to undertake this in two or three stages). Like others, Strauss was concerned about the deleterious effects of an ileostomy. In his young patient, Koenig, he at last found an individual equipped to deal with the problems, for Koenig was a chemistry student with a flair for mechanics and of an artistic inclination. Koenig had to have an ileostomy and he needed little encouragement from Strauss to pursue the idea of designing a bag to collect the excreta; a bag which could be stuck to the skin, which would not leak and so would prevent any soiling of skin and undergarments. Under Strauss' guidance Koenig came up with the solution – a rubber pouch so slender as to be indiscernible even under tight fitting garments and a glue to stick this to the skin.

In 1947 a few samples were brought to England by a Midlands physician, Lionel Hardy, who had many colitic patients under his care, and there in Birmingham he set me to work to try the appliances out. It was first necessary to develop a stoma best suited to the adherent bag and the surgical technique to achieve a good fit so that the result would be free of complications. This done, it was obvious that the appliance had much to offer; however, further supplies became difficult to obtain, restricted as we were at that time as regards the availability of foreign currency and in particular, dollars. Despite a threat from the American manufacturer that we would be infringing his patent we proceeded to arrange the manufacture in Birmingham of the appliance and the cement, which on analysis in the chemistry department of the university proved to be no more nor less than latex solution as used in puncture mending outfits, laced with zinc oxide to give it a suitably medicinal appearance.

Almost overnight the outlook in this depressing, disabling and not uncommonly fatal disease had changed. Ulcerative colitis is confined to the large intestine; the large intestine is disposable; a patient is restored to normal weight and health when irreparably damaged bowel is removed. With an efficient ileostomy controlled by an adherent appliance a patient can return to normal life and normal activity. No recreation, pastime or sport, no form of work is denied to him or her. The young woman can have a baby; the child can go to school; a man can take up his job, the businessman at his desk, the miner in the pit. For the Koenig bag remains sealed to the skin for days at a time, upwards of a week, after which it is changed, its contents being emptied at convenient moments during the day.

*

The adherent bag changed the outcome because it enabled damaged bowel to be removed as a matter of choice. Ulcerative colitis is a disease of the young starting mostly in the early years of life. Before 1944 few patients were likely to make old bones; now, following recovery from the operation necessary to remove the large bowel, life returns to normal in quality and duration. I know patients upon whom I operated thirty years and more ago, now enjoying retirement after a fully active life. The operation itself is not a serious one, the risk of dying as a result could hardly be lower being no greater than one per cent. Though the same cannot be said of the emergency situation: when the bowel begins to disintegrate and operation has to go ahead perforce under very unfavourable circumstances, because the condition has run out of medical control and the risk of persisting with it is even greater than recourse to surgery. By then matters are out of hand. There are signs to indicate when disintegration is on the verge of occurring; armed with this anticipation it is possible to remove the colon before it becomes hazardous to do so.

Ironically, the very success brought about by the advent of a manageable stoma has led to attempts to dispense with it. Once it became evident that removal of the bowel was an effective treatment for ulcerative colitis it was not unreasonable to argue that a similar result could be achieved by removing all but the last few inches of the rectum so that a junction could be formed by anastomosis between it and the ileum, thus dispensing with a stoma altogether. But despite maintaining anal function in this way the benefits have proved somewhat illusory, more apparent than real. Patients with ileo-rectal anastomosis seldom open their bowels less than four times a day and not infrequently more often; control can be imperfect because of looseness of the motion and the precipitant sense of urgency which besets the patient until it is passed. Moreover the retention of even so small a fringe of abnormal bowel can invoke any of the complications of ulcerative colitis: trouble in joints, in the skin and in the eyes, and even the high risk of cancer developing later. It has become clear that total ablation of large bowel and nothing less is needed to cure the disease. None would deny that to have an ileostomy is to endure an imperfection. Nevertheless it is a comparatively small price to pay for the return to normal health and a full life.

But might it not be possible to devise an ileostomy which dispenses with the need for a bag to control it? After perfecting the method in dogs, Neils Kock, a Swede, put this idea into practice in 1968 fashioning a reservoir from ileum to provide a receptacle for faeces within the abdomen with an outlet flush on the abdominal wall which could be emptied from time to time by passing a catheter. The technique is ingenious but complex; in effect something like the old-fashioned unspillable inkwell is constructed by joining together adjacent loops of ileum, opening them into one another to form a single cavity and invaginating the outflow from this by pushing it back and fixing it – not a procedure to be undertaken lightly by anyone but an expert in the field and not a general purpose operation within the compass of every surgeon. Although it does not confer the advantage of anal control, here was an enterprising step forwards; nevertheless it is still limited in application because of yet unresolved complications. It is all too easy for the invaginated 'nipple' to unravel within a year or two so that a further operation has to be undertaken in about a third of those possessing this pouch, in order to restore the continence it is designed to confer. Continence is, in effect, achieved by reliance upon obstruction to the passage of intestinal contents; although this is intermittent, evidence is accumulating that it may sometimes have deleterious consequences in the long term.

More promising may be a rather different application of this idea developed by Parks in London. The reservoir is similarly constructed from adjacent segments of ileum; these are placed in the pelvis and attached to the anus after all of the large intestine has been removed including the rectum, except for the lowermost part of its muscular wall through which the ileum is pulled down to the anus. By this means it is intended to preserve something akin to the sensation we ordinarily feel in the pelvis with the need to defaecate. Anal function is thus restored without the imperfections which follow a direct attachment of ileum to rectum and, possibly, with fewer complications than are encountered with the continent ileostomy. But, like Kock's reservoir, this also needs the test of time before a proper assessment can be made. All is not yet perfect, but in terms

109

of development of an operation these are early days; it would be a mistake to think that normal bowel control is automatically conferred by operation. Continence is for the most part achieved, although about one third of patients with the pelvic contrivance wear a pad for safety usually at night, and a catheter is used by half the patients to empty the reservoir. Another difficulty can occur which does not affect to any appreciable degree those with a Kock's pouch. In one in ten the skin round the anus becomes sore; around the abdominal opening of a Kock's pouch this rarely happens. What can be said about both devices is that they are excellent when all goes well but that they are not yet one hundred per cent proof against breakdown.

*

Koenig's invention of an adherent bag and the perfection of a simple outlet to match it started a revolution in more ways than one. It placed an operation to remove the large bowel on the map as an effective means of eliminating ulcerative colitis; it turned urological minds to the construction of a urinary conduit which would provide control by similar means; it made doctors think again about the time-honoured colostomy, the care and management of which had been neglected. An adherent appliance is a neat way of covering and protecting a colostomy even though it cannot contain solid large bowel excreta.

In addition individuals with a stoma began to take a part in the medical and surgical matters which affected them. For who can know best how to control a stoma? Not the doctor, who can only surmise what difficulties may have to be dealt with in the course of a normal day; nor the nurse who likewise can only guess at the problems. So it fell to the ileostomists themselves to pioneer the ways and means, to lay down the guidelines, to discover the intricacies of effective adherence and of skin care around the stoma. Not just because they were the 'consumers', nor simply because they alone and not the doctor, surgeon or nurse had first hand experience. But because in the management of an ileostomy success is complete, failure utter; there are no grey areas of compromise enabling an ileostomist to get away with it. If the appliance can be made to work the individual with an ileostomy can do anything; if it does not he or she is seriously disabled.

In Birmingham when we first embarked upon surgery for the treatment of ulcerative colitis and I began to feel my way as regards fashioning an ileostomy to fit the bag, we were faced with the problem that nobody had had experience in the matter – neither physician, surgeon, nurse nor patient. In those pioneering days all four became united in an intimate group; we on the medical side soon began to learn from our patients. Meanwhile Dr Lionel Hardy had struck upon a bright idea to comfort the patients faced with the daunting prospect of an operation which would leave them with an artificial opening on the front of the belly for life. The idea seems obvious now for it has been adopted worldwide: he simply invited someone with an established ileostomy to visit any new candidate for operation. He had two purposes in mind. First, the visitor, restored to health, vigour and a normal life, provided a living demonstration to the prostrate, wasted, debilitated patient of the recovery at his command, of what was on offer in return for the price of a permanent ileostomy. Furthermore this provided the prospective ileostomist with a friend at court to answer any question however intimate, a friend who could be believed more certainly than the reassuring doctor or nurse. Gradually a group of men and women of varying age, ability and standing were gathered together, all of them willing to undertake this voluntary task. Very effective they have proved to be as visitors still are, the world over; for the practice of visiting in this way has become a cardinal principle of stoma care whatever the stoma may be. But standards vary so it is not always put into practice.

The next problem which fell to our lot was how to instruct patients when they came to leave hospital, how to provide them with all the information they would require to keep them going after they returned home, indeed how to anticipate those unforeseen needs which must necessarily vary from one individual to another. It would take time, often up to an hour or more, to explain to patients how to contend with difficulty after the support of the ward and the training and experience given by staff had been withdrawn. So in 1955 a development came about new to the British scene: an association was started by patients for patients. It is true that there was already in existence at least one such society for patients, the Diabetic Association, but this had been set up by doctors for patients, originally to facilitate the distribution of insulin to diabetics.

The Ileostomy Association of Great Britain and Ireland was founded by patients – by a particular patient in fact. Doreen Harris, who had been one of the first of our hospital visitors, suggested to me that the time had come for those with an ileostomy to meet, since their number was now rising notably and there should be matters of mutual interest which could be discussed to the advantage of all. This was the moment we on the medical side had been waiting for; we had not wished to establish an association ourselves thinking it more likely that it would thrive and become more effective if founded on 'customer' demand. And so it has proved for it is flourishing today and more effectively than ever.

The nucleus was formed by those hospital visitors enrolled by Lionel Hardy; the organisation of visiting, and the selection and training of visitors was their primary role and I was happy to pass to them the supervision and support of the new ileostomist in the home. We doctors did not withdraw completely; the members of the IA were going to need our support in dealing with the profession generally (which needed to be educated as we had been about the care of stoma patients), with hospitals, with the retailers and manufacturers of appliances and adhesives, and to be guided through the tricky minefields of medical ethics. The horizons soon widened; the Association was able to give information and make suggestions to improve manufacturers' products; new and more convenient appliances and adhesives were developed at the instigation of the Association. Training films were made, mutual support given; IA began to take over the role of a pressure group in the best possible sense, *vis à vis* the Department of Health, the Ministry of Health as it then was.

112

It was unique and it was successful; hardly surprising, therefore, that another association like it for those with artificial outlets for urine, the Urinary Conduit Association, was founded fifteen years later on very similar lines. The Colostomy Welfare Group – the name speaks for itself – has come into being more recently and is rather different in nature. It has no membership other than the volunteers who participate in its visiting service; it is run by a council of medical men. The reason for the difference must be obvious when one considers that colostomy is nearly always the outcome of an operation undertaken for removal of a cancer.

In the United States similar associations began to appear rather earlier than IA. In such a vast continent they were perforce based upon cities, whereas IA was a national organisation from the moment, six months or so after Doreen Harris' first moves in the Midlands, when similar developments took place in London. Thereafter IA spread over the country from a Birmingham–London axis. In the USA, Boston was one of the first, if not the first city to establish an association, as was New York; QT Boston it was called because at that time American ileostomists and colostomists (both being included in membership) felt that the possession of a stoma made them outcasts from society. It was better for the information to be 'on the QT', a phrase older readers will recall as meaning on the quiet. While Americans sought to conceal their identity, British ileostomists took the opposite view; they felt that the possession of a stoma should not be treated in covert fashion since this was to condone the attitude that a stoma was more a disgrace than a disability. It was their opinion that by education alone would public opinion change from an attitude of rejection to acceptance of those who, through no fault of their own, but by misfortune found themselves having to face life with a stoma. American opinion has changed; from QT they have become Ostomy Associations, each group in the North American continent being linked in the United Ostomy Association, while aspirations world wide are being achieved biennially at meetings of delegates from ostomy associations throughout the world under the aegis of the International Ostomy Association.

Part of the revolution which has followed the successful establishment of ileostomy has been the recent institution of a new field of nursing care, the speciality of stoma care. It started in 1969 at the Cleveland Clinic USA from a suggestion made by a surgeon, Rupert Turnbull, to one of his patients with a successful ileostomy, Norma Gill, that she should advise stoma patients who came to see him in his clinic. Norma Gill, who was not a registered nurse, made a study of the problems she encountered there and set about resolving them; she then began to train others in what Rupert Turnbull called enterostomal therapy. Enterostomal therapy is now a recognised occupation for which a diploma of ET is awarded.

In the UK the approach has been somewhat different. At a rather earlier date the Ileostomy Association had responded to the request for experienced volunteers to come forward to assist in hospital clinics; this was undertaken on a small scale in areas with a special interest in stoma care. At the same time appliance manufacturers, sensing the need among their clientele for sound practical advice, began to employ experienced ileostomists in clinics of their own. Meanwhile the Ileostomy Association, which had been organising short courses for nurses and other interested parties, began to prevail upon the Department of Health to consider special training courses for registered nurses and to create posts for stoma care nurses, who although based upon hospitals could also go out into the community and attend patients in their homes.

The stoma care nurse has become a specialist who has gained knowledge and experience in a recondite field; her role is expanding in interesting ways. Because of the problems inherent in the application of a bag and what failure may bring in its train she has become an expert in skin care, so that her assistance may now be sought in the management of pressure sores and excoriation associated with incontinence to be seen in the elderly, the infirm and the bed-ridden. Rather more surprising is her emergence as a sex counsellor. Men are prepared to broach the subject and put problems they may have in this respect to her, because few inhibitions remain between a patient and the nurse who deals with his stoma. Natural reticence is overcome by this innocent intimacy.

8 Crohn's disease

The story of ulcerative colitis has changed radically during this century – indeed virtually during the brief period since World War II – from gloom to success, with the emphasis passing from medicine to surgery. Over the almost identical period the story of Crohn's disease has likewise altered fundamentally, but in exactly the opposite direction, from what appeared to be success to gloom, the emphasis passing from surgery to medicine. How has this come about?

Cast your mind back to 1932 and imagine the impact of Dr Crohn's revelations. Here was a localised area of inflammation confined to the last few inches or so of the terminal ileum. The abnormality and its site could not have been better designed for surgical removal or, to make the job even simpler, for bypass. The small intestine, so nicely placed, so accessible and mobile in the central area of the abdomen is easy to operate upon, unless inflammation has plastered together adjacent loops of small intestine to present a difficulty which adds spice for a surgeon to an otherwise straightforward operation to remove the lesion, or which, for the timorous, can be overcome by making a short circuit. The loss of a segment of lower ileum was at that time considered to be of little consequence since digestion and absorption was thought to be complete by the time the contents of the gut reached that area.

Unknown to medicine then were the details of vitamin B, indeed of vitamins in general since they were in the process of being discovered. We now know more, in particular that there is more than one vitamin B, and that this group regulates the formation of red blood corpuscles. Two forms of the vitamin are of particular importance when it comes to removing parts of the stomach or small intestine. A persistent dearth of folic acid depletes the red cells of haemoglobin, so vital in transporting oxygen, thus inducing anaemia; disease in the upper reaches of the gut can bring this about, as can surgical removal of any sizeable area. Anaemia in another form ensues when the last part of the ileum is removed. Vitamin B_{12}, cyanocobalamin, is absorbed in that area and the amount which may be removed by operation or be rendered useless by disease is critically limited. Thus a form of anaemia with a reduced number of red cells mostly larger than usual but each carrying rather more haemoglobin than they should but insufficient in total, is likely to develop slowly as stores of cyanocobalamin in the liver get used up.

Almost daily we learn of some new intestinal function, shedding a little further light upon those dark recesses. It is not so long ago that the area of absorption of vitamin B_{12} became linked with that of bile salts; when the last part of the ileum is put out of action by disease or taken out by operation they too lose the area necessary for their absorption. Two physiological disturbances follow with diarrhoea as a result; the first concerns bile conservation. The complex bile salts are ordinarily retained in the body, being returned to the liver from the ileum to be poured out again higher up so as to emulsify the fats ready for digestion as they enter the duodenum. Disruption of this circulating pool of bile salts impairs the assimilation of fats and so can lead to diarrhoea through fat excretion. Furthermore as these bile salts leak onwards through into the colon bacterial colonisation there is disturbed; diarrhoea ensues.

So removal of intestine, a bit here and a bit there, is less innocuous than was thought in the days before the war. This comprehension is recent, and no doubt greater understanding will follow to underline the truism that no part of our anatomy should be considered redundant. Evolution results in the ultimate in efficiency since it makes use of anything to hand to equip us for the great struggle while eradicating whatever becomes redundant. Even the appendix, I suspect, will be found to fulfill some better purpose than providing a simple training ground for aspiring surgeons.

But to return to 1932: here for the surgeon was a god-send, a well-circumscribed swelling which no doctor could dispel with physic. Here was an inflammatory mass, not a cancer. Until then tuberculosis had been thought to be the sole cause of ileitis; tuberculous ileitis could not be cured by operation. The sight of Crohn's ileitis made surgical fingers itch; the only trouble being the rarity of a lesion which permitted surgeons the pleasure of a satisfactory operation and the gratifying prospect of a cure. So few and far between were these cases that optimism in the outcome prevailed for twenty years or more and only began to decline as more cases accumulated and continued to be studied over a number of years.

It was not however the surgically inflicted anaemia or diarrhoea which brought on the era of therapeutic pessimism. Folic acid absorption can be enhanced by giving it in tablets instead of relying upon natural provision in food; cyanocobalamin depots in the liver can be restored by injection. Even the diarrhoea can be mitigated, though not always, by ingesting a special resin designed to mop up the bile salts and render them harmless.

The first set-back was recurrence; recurrence can mean different things, as will be seen. First it became obvious that although activity in the form of symptoms usually subsided after a bypass operation they soon and inevitably returned; hardly surprising, since the area involved in Crohn's disease had not been removed. All this only proved that 'resting' the area in the sense of diverting intestinal contents away from the inflammation and ulceration conferred no lasting effect. This situation should be regarded more as reactivation than recurrence. For some inexplicable reason 'reactivation' is a term infrequently used in this context, a reflection perhaps of a disinclination within medicine for semantic accuracy. Not infrequently the inflammation progressed despite the bypass, albeit more quietly, to abscess and even fistula formation. The bypass operation has fallen into disuse except when it is thought that operative difficulty may otherwise arise.

Removal of the area of ileitis is a different matter; this would appear to eliminate the disease but it does not. The condition reappears sooner or later at the site where the ends of the intestine were joined together in anastomosis after the affected portion had been removed. Here at least is recurrence of the original lesion. From 1960 onwards, thirty years after Crohn's original description, we began to be aware of the tendency for this to happen, though not always with doleful effect since x-rays may sometimes show an anastomotic recurrence which is not causing symptoms. In addition time has disclosed something of greater concern to us: lesions develop at new sites despite the elimination of the original one – yet another form of recurrence. To make matters worse we now know that recurrence in whatever sense we choose to use the term is inevitable. Recurrence will have presented itself in 30 to 50 per cent of patients submitted to operation five years previously; after 10 to 15 years the number rises to 80 per cent.

*

Where else does Crohn's disease become manifest? Not only around the orifices; from time to time it can affect the skin in situations remote from mouth or anus although this is as rare as Crohn's ulceration of the gullet or stomach. This universality, the fact that the whole of the gut is at risk, has only recently been acknowledged. In those distant days in Birmingham when we began to develop the surgery appropriate for ulcerative colitis, we observed certain types of colitis which did not fit the pattern of ulcerative colitis. In some there were clear indications of Crohn's lesions in the small intestine; not unnaturally we regarded the colitis in such cases as being of Crohn's origin and labelled them as such. Elsewhere the view was taken that ulcerative colitis and Crohn's disease were coexistent, and that all cases which presented only with colitis were *ipso facto* ulcerative colitis whether or not they fitted the accepted pattern of that disease.

For a number of years controversy persisted, very rightly so since a proper understanding of disease develops through discussion. Physicians in the USA persisted in regarding any and every case of colitis as ulcerative colitis despite good microscopical evidence presented from London supporting our contention that some cases fell into the category of Crohn's disease. By the end of the 1960s there was general agreement throughout the world that Crohn's disease does affect the large bowel though it starts there rather less frequently than it does in the ileum. Ironically the last centre to concede this point was Mount Sinai Hospital and Dr Crohn himself.

The implications of this have had a profound effect. If the whole of the intestine is at risk does this indicate that even at the outset the gut is in some way abnormal throughout its length despite there being only one obvious area of abnormality to be seen? If so, the prospect of halting the disease by removal of the presenting lesion, in the way that we may sometimes catch cancer in the nick of time before it has spread, is a concept doomed to failure. Indeed, is Crohn's disease inexorable, more so in a way than cancer? Although recurrence in Crohn's disease is inevitable it does not share with cancer the facility to spread itself by injecting malignant cells into the blood stream to get going again at other sites in the body.

So surgery is no longer the first option; has it any place in Crohn's disease? In the strategy of management of a disease clearly cure is the prime objective; more and more as the twentieth century has progressed the disclosures of science have enabled us to achieve this. But when this desirable aim proves elusive we are by no means powerless; if a disease cannot be eliminated its effects may be mitigated or brought under control and held in check. Indeed this discretion is sometimes the better part of therapeutic valour as has already been observed in certain circumstances of food poisoning: better to sway with the wind until the storm has passed rather than run the risk of counter-attack by bacteria made resistant to antibiotics by our imperfect attempts to eliminate them.

119

But this could never be said of a disease where we still remain ignorant of its cause; only when the cause becomes known will we be in a position to choose. This must apply to Crohn's disease; even when it is known what lies behind the condition there may be no immediate antidote. The management of Crohn's disease is very like the situation in tuberculosis up to thirty years ago before specific and effective drugs were discovered to eliminate the tubercle bacillus. The coincidence does not stop there for Crohn's disease simulates tuberculosis in numerous other ways, not least in a similarity to be observed under the microscope.

In keeping with many other chronic disorders tuberculosis varies in activity so that at times, often during long periods, a patient would be well and able to participate in ordinary daily life, apart, perhaps, from energetic pursuits; at others he or she would be incapacitated by malaise and more specific symptoms, particularly coughing when the lungs were affected as they most often were. During these periods of relapse recourse was had to very general means of support, which used to be aimed on the one hand at 'building up the body's defences', on the other at easing symptoms. So the patient would be made to rest in bed to allow, it was thought, the body's strength to be conserved and directed towards healing, a nebulous and unexplained concept if ever there was one. The fact that the disease tended naturally to fluctuate between activity and remission was perhaps disregarded; the benefit contributed by enforced rest was never put to the test of a controlled trial (the method employed today to resolve such dilemmas by comparing a group under treatment with a similar group suffering from the same condition but not receiving that treatment).

It was all too obvious that a broken bone would not heal if the affected limb was not kept at rest, to the extent even of splinting it; and so with other injuries. By analogy the lungs should be put at rest as far as possible to permit them to heal and, more generally though less realistically, the body should be rested so that its defences could be concentrated upon healing: a time-honoured concept, which still tempers therapeutic attitudes today particularly towards chronic disease, although it is difficult to conceive how recumbency and inertia can have any direct effect upon those small cells whose function is defence through their ability to produce substances capable of counteracting microorganisms and their toxins. While it cannot be denied that rest may be of general benefit this has yet to be proved.

But bed rest brings benefit in other ways. A patient lying in bed has to be looked after; food has to be brought regularly to him. Fever is associated with weight loss partly because of an increased need for energy to sustain the higher temperature (as with any mechanical heater), and this is only forthcoming if food intake is increased. More often than not a sick person is 'off his food'; hence loss of weight through failure to meet increased need is further compounded by reduced intake. Despite the old adage – feed a cold starve a fever – there is a need for the chronically ill to take more food. The patient who has to remain in bed has to have meals brought to him so he comes under a watchful eye and food is presented to him at regular intervals. He should not lose by default calories he needs.

Bed rest, improved nutrition and moderation of symptoms have again become the first line of treatment in a chronic disease, now that experience has shown that Crohn's disease cannot be eliminated by operation and we are confronted by circumstances not dissimilar to phthisis. Instead of a chronic cough the major symptom is diarrhoea; malaise, loss of weight, anaemia and chronic infection are symptoms common to both illnesses. There is also the occasional abscess discharging persistently, in Crohn's disease as a fistula, in tuberculosis often as persistent sputum though sometimes fistulously. So the strategy of treatment in Crohn's disease has moved perforce from elimination of the disease to attempting to modify its manifestations as was the policy for tuberculosis in the pre-antibiotic era. Here is a disease of ups and downs so why not boost the ups and thus endeavour to encourage a remission to take place?

Hence the need for bed rest when the going gets tough and symptoms deteriorate. This simple measure often has the immediate effect of calming diarrhoea; the bowels open less frequently and the stools improve, an effect which can be enhanced by simple drugs like codeine phosphate or more modern pharmaceutical developments specifically designed for the purpose like loperamide and diphenoxylate. As added benefit abdominal pain begins to subside. Since this symptom tends to manifest itself soon after eating has begun it is a potent deterrent to taking food and so contributes to loss of weight. Appetite is not lost, however, so the relief of pain restores the desire to eat. When weight starts to be gained a remission is on the way.

If, because of a fistula, weight loss inexorably continues we now have another method of restoring calorie balance from loss to gain by feeding fats, amino-acids and sugars into a vein, and this can be continued over prolonged periods. With improved nutrition and with the intestines completely at rest the fistula can close. Moreover it is no longer necessary for the patient to stay in hospital while receiving such treatment. A small operation allows a special little valve to be inserted into a vein and through this the patient can run in liquid nourishment at home, appropriate in amount and supplied in bottles from the hospital. This provides release from bondage in more ways than one, for as strength is regained a return can be made to daily activities including work; the fistulous discharge is much reduced since no food has to enter the gut to be digested, and so it remains until the fistula closes of its own accord. Pregnancy has now been achieved and brought to a successful conclusion in these circumstances.

*

Drugs may help, particularly steroids though their effect of increasing weight has nothing permanent about it; this occurs because steroids cause water to be retained in the body. They came into use for no better reason than by analogy with ulcerative colitis. They are the first choice for they not infrequently get a remission going and they also create a sense of wellbeing and improve the appetite.

Whether they have any more specific effect on the disease it is hard to say. Weight loss is a cardinal sign of activity of the disease; put this into reverse and a remission is on its way. In fact a plethora of drugs is used because no single one is reliable. The response to any one drug may be good but it is unpredictable; it may ease the condition of one person and yet not suit another. To give an example: in 1967 when beginning to despair of the effectiveness of surgery in certain cases, and in particular in one young man whose disease recurred repeatedly with intestinal fistulation after operations designed to eradicate it and who was at death's door, I resorted in desperation to a drug which had not previously been used for patients with Crohn's disease. It was an immunosuppressive drug called azathioprine: the choice came about like this.

The distinguishing mark of Crohn's disease already described, the so-called granuloma, presents a distinctive ring of white cells, lymphocytes, around the periphery. Those cells participate in reactions which bring about protection through immunity. Sometimes they can be a nuisance: as in certain conditions when the immune reaction turns against us, or more accurately against tissues which are part of us. Autoimmune disease takes various forms. It is exemplified by transplantation of an organ like a kidney from one individual to another, even more so when an attempt is made from one species to another. The kidney will be rejected by the immune reaction, and the lymphocytes play a dominant role in bringing this about. Before kidney transplantation could get under way means had to be found to counteract this reaction. Attempts were made to promote an antiserum against lymphocytes. This was developed in the same way that antiserum has always been developed, as against diphtheria and other toxins, of tetanus and typhoid for instance by raising the antiserum in horses.

Sometimes the immune process, which for the most part protects us, turns against us. The thyroid is a particular tissue which can trigger off an autoimmune reaction. Under viral attack it can be damaged in a way which causes its

123

own special globulin, to which is attached thyroxin the active hormone which the gland provides, to leak out beyond the confines of the gland itself. The globulin brings immunity into play and the outcome is persistent inflammation and ultimate replacement of the thyroid by nondescript scar tissue. In many ways the reaction of Crohn's disease resembles the inflammation which destroys the thyroid. So why not try to reverse the reaction and what better way to achieve this than antilymphocytic serum which was in use at that time to keep graft rejection at bay?

This was the reasoning that set the path to immunosuppression for Crohn's disease. I drew a blank in my attempts to obtain the serum; it was in short supply at the time, under strict control and distributed on an establishment network committed to kidney transplantation, to whom the use I proposed must have seemed ôutré. This failure though irritating at the time proved a blessing in disguise since the serum later fell into disuse because it could not be purified of all sensitising matter; moreover I was forced to consider other drugs coming onto the market for immunosuppression, and chose azathioprine.

To my surprise the young man did not die, then to my disbelief began to improve; the fistulas healed and he became well. With this encouragement, it was natural to proceed further; six other cases previously intractable to all forms of treatment in use at that time, responded well. Yet this was no breakthrough; by a quirk of fortune six successive patients recovered and their recovery was maintained while they continued to take azathioprine. But the luck did not hold; as the drug came to be used more and more it was obvious that while some patients responded remarkably others remained untouched; it was impossible to predict from the clinical features of each case which patient would respond, which would not.

That is how matters stand today. The effectiveness of azathioprine has been studied widely here and more extensively in the USA in controlled trials which have failed to provide statistical proof that azathioprine is more effective than a dummy pill. So why continue to give it? The answer is that although its effect in individual cases can be considerable, this may take place too infrequently and too unpredictably to produce a significant change in statistics culled from large numbers. Herein lies a weakness of clinical trials, more particularly when the result is non-committal. Conclusions drawn from large numbers sometimes indicate little where an individual is concerned.

Nearly twenty years later, it transpires that the effectiveness of azathioprine is probably due less to immunosuppression than to its anti-inflammatory properties. Or because, as has now been shown, it acts like an antibiotic against anaerobic bacteria, of which many varieties exist in the gut where their presence can prevent ulcers healing. All of which emphasises the unpredictability of drugs in the treatment of Crohn's disease.

Because it has proved of value in ulcerative colitis it is understandable that sulphasalazine should be prescribed for Crohn's colitis, but as with steroids improvement is less obvious in Crohn's disease. The picture is the reverse of that seen with azathioprine; some improvement takes place with the sulpha drug sufficiently often to score statistically although in the individual case it has scant effect.

The multiplication of drugs in use is evidence of our therapeutic impotence. When one drug fails we try another; there is no single compound to be relied upon with certainty to promote a remission. At the next flare up success may not be repeated with the medicine used on the first occasion; another has to be found. Hence the need always to have another shot in the locker. And in contrast to ulcerative colitis, there is no drug which will prevent symptoms recurring in a patient with quiescent disease; neither sulphasalazine nor steroids are effective in this way.

*

To return to the question posed earlier: now that we know that Crohn's disease cannot be eliminated even by removal of the obvious abnormality with wide margins of more normal gut on either side – a contention which was being made for a time – is there any need for operation at all? To that question the answer is unhesitatingly yes. A patient may need more support when the disease is active than medical care has to offer; circumstances can arise which call for operation. An abscess may develop in one of several areas and require drainage, on the abdominal wall or beside the anus; it could burst and drain of its own accord but it is often better lanced in anticipation of this in order to relieve pain.

That little operation sets further problems; or, to be more exact, the draining abscess does: for it now represents a fistula, that is an outlet from the intestine onto the skin with the potential to discharge gut contents there, though at first this may not be obvious while pus alone is being discharged. The abscess develops because Crohn's ulceration within the gut gradually erodes its way through the wall to break out of its intestinal confines; so when the abscess cavity drains onto the surface it also has a communication into the intestinal canal on its dark undisclosed side. The course the fistula takes is not a direct straight line, between A and B as it were; its very tortuosity can deny access to bowel contents. But if the gut beyond is much narrowed by the disease the chance of diversion of faeces along the fistula is greater.

Hence the intermittency with which a fistula reveals itself; as likely as not it will be active for a few days at a time, then cease to eject anything but pus, cruelly raising hope that it may be closing, only to erupt again. Hope should not be entirely dashed by this for when remission comes a fistula, if it is going to heal, does not do so pronto, overnight; the periods without discharge get longer while the days marked by a discharge become fewer and further between, until they cease. That is the pattern when azathioprine proves effective, though instead of taking one to two months or more it is speeded up into an equivalent period of weeks. A fistula does not respond directly to steroid treatment, though that may invoke a remission which ultimately brings on its closure.

Circumstances are rather different when the intestine

becomes narrowed so much as to begin to obstruct the passage of its contents at the point beyond where the fistula starts. Here is a mechanical situation which makes it unlikely that the fistula will close. At this juncture an operation is needed to overcome the obstruction by the simple process of removing the narrow area taking with it for good measure the fistula itself.

Anal fistulas are better not removed because the surgical wound which results remains indolently and resolutely unhealed, in contrast to what happens after an operation for simple fistula not arising from Crohn's disease. But they can sometimes be improved. If a stricture inside the back passage is obstructing and so tending to deflect faeces down the fistula outside the control of the valve-like sphincter to cause incontinence and soiling, simple dilatation may bring about wonders.

That process of ulceration causing penetration through the intestinal wall could theoretically lead to perforation with intestinal contents flowing freely into the peritoneal cavity, which is only a potential cavity designed to harbour and protect the gut and other abdominal organs. This would be a serious matter for generalised peritonitis would follow, as it does when a stomach or duodenal ulcer, the common cause of indigestion, perforates.

Here is a situation of emergency which develops but rarely in Crohn's disease, remarkable as that may seem in view of the extensive areas which can be involved. But Crohn's ulceration usually progresses at a snail-like pace, allowing reaction to occur and adhesions to form to bind loops of intestine together and generally close up the oncoming breach in a variety of ways. The adherence of one loop to another may encourage an internal fistula between them but this is often of little account except when it creates a wide short circuit with baneful effects on nutrition, an unwelcome event easily corrected by operation.

The emergency brought about by perforation and leakage directly into the abdominal cavity calls for immediate operation. On the whole, emergency operations have to be undertaken rarely in Crohn's disease, the risk of perforation being not more than one in a hundred cases. Acute and severe bleeding from a blood vessel which suddenly gives way through being exposed in the base of an ulcer is no more common, probably less so; but the urgency of operation to close the leak is greater since much blood can be lost in a short time. Another risk when ulceration of the large bowel goes too far is the weakness which may develop causing general disintegration of its wall; this can happen in Crohn's disease as in ulcerative colitis, and with any other state of persistent ulceration, like ischaemic colitis – in any form of colitis in fact. Removal of the colon becomes a matter of urgency not only because the bowel wall may give way with the same dire result as perforation, but also because of the toxic effects inseparable from that state.

In the main, surgery for Crohn's disease is a deliberate affair undertaken at a moment of choice, convenient to the patient and all concerned, because it is part of a programme of support, and is in principle inseparable from medical care. In a word: its purpose is palliation. The main symptoms of pain and diarrhoea may defy the beneficial effects of rest and settling drugs so that easement can only be obtained by resorting to removal of that part of the bowel which is most affected. This is particularly so when the pain is of that gripping, intermittent colicky nature which presages obstruction. In these circumstances, though relief may be obtained by going to bed for a day or two, it may not be long-lived, so that the area narrowed by the scarring which results from longstanding ulceration has to be taken away sooner rather than later.

In the young there are other rather more pressing reasons for operation. Often a child fails to thrive, growth becomes retarded and puberty is delayed; thus a teenage patient becomes underweight, short of stature and physically immature. Unless something is done early enough things will go too far and go on for too long to allow reversal of these negative trends. If action is taken in time and an area of active ileitis is removed a remission will follow which will permit a young patient to get back on course; all the height which has been lost can be recovered before another bout of active disease intervenes, and with luck adulthood may have been reached by then. So in these limited circumstances operation will take precedence as soon as it is seen that full relief is not being obtained by less radical means.

*

Earlier it was stated that recurrence follows operation within five years in half those previously operated upon. One question is not infrequently asked by patients or their relations: do symptoms recur at ever more frequent intervals? If anything, the reverse is true: as time goes on the periods between attacks get longer. A further question: how often does one operation lead to another? Looking back over the last thirty years at five hundred or more patients treated in Birmingham it seems that, on the average, in patients having to undergo surgery on the small bowel for the first time at about 25 years old there is a fifty fifty chance that 15 years will pass before another operation is needed; most will have to submit to surgery between twice or three times in their lifetime.

*

One other reason for operation remains – the need to find out what really is wrong. An Asian woman with symptoms of gut trouble whose x-rays show abnormality in the small intestine just like Crohn's disease: has she got Crohn's disease or tuberculous ileitis which can be indistinguishable from it? The answer may be unobtainable without taking a look inside the abdomen at the intestine itself and possibly obtaining samples of tissue to be examined under a microscope. That is not the only condition which may mimic Crohn's disease; nevertheless an operation to establish a diagnosis is not a common event. It is rather more common, perhaps, for the abdomen to be opened on a misapprehension, because what turns out to be Crohn's disease was thought to be some other condition necessitating immediate operation. Acute ileitis is a case in point; it can easily be revealed as an embarrassment to a young surgeon who has got up in the middle of the night expecting to remove an inflamed appendix.

PART THREE
A frustrating search

9 Chronic diarrhoea: seeking the cause

Do we ever know the cause of a disease? There are times when this seems doubtful, for even when some noxious agent is identified there still remains the question as to why or how it struck. We are content when we learn that an attack of diarrhoea can be attributed to the presence of, say, shigella in the gut and are less concerned with how it came to be around making one man sick but not the next. Looked at the other way, there would certainly have been no diarrhoea if the organism had not been around. So shigella was the causative agent though there were other circumstances paving the way to the illness which it was capable of creating. In a sense the problem is philosophical; but for those who have to treat the sick it is none the less practical.

Aetiology is the word used in medicine to cover these numerous and nebulous phenomena which contribute to the disease. Nor is an understanding of the aetiological factors involved in a particular condition just an academic exercise designed to titilate the interest of doctors. Before specific antibiotics were developed for tuberculosis, treatment was based in part upon mitigation of the aetiological factors whenever this was possible and in whatever way feasible. They carry little weight in treatment when there is an effective antidote to the main cause; that is why antibiotics which home in on their targets with such accuracy that illness is nipped in the bud have altered the scene so radically. The emphasis on aetiology is all the greater when the main cause of a disease is unknown, the more so because it represents the milieu in which that central cause can operate. Recognition of antecedents and determinants may present clues which can assist in its recognition. So it is that in the absence of any obvious cause for ulcerative colitis or Crohn's disease, interest has been inclined to concentrate upon their aetiology.

It will come as no surprise that medical fashions in vogue at any one time tend to be reflected in the aetiological

133

factors. After the collapse of Bargen's bacillus as the contender for the doubtful honour of being the *fons et origo* of ulcerative colitis earlier this century (Dr Bargen of the Mayo Clinic had published his report in 1924) attention began to be concentrated upon stress and the psycho-soma. Stress has long been considered to be injurious to man and in the absence of any evidence to the contrary it continues so, despite the lack of evidence to support the assumption. Maybe the 'surges of adrenalin' so beloved of the modern novelist and thriller writer, when they actually occur do represent a harmful response, albeit a proper and natural one; again there is no evidence to support the implication unless the individual under stress is already suffering from raised blood pressure. Stress is invoked to be condemned as injurious only because it flatters the ego, on the same premise that we can *suffer* from overwork, and that this lies at the root of such disasters as coronary thrombosis. The only harm in the myth of stress as a cause of disease lies in the degree to which it can hoodwink doctors; in various insidious ways it does.

In the late 1940s and for the next ten years psychosomatic disease came very much into vogue; the thought that psychological disorder, or even the normal mind, could alter the substantial body in such a way as to lead to organic disease with physical changes discernible under the microscope, held many attractions, not least of which was the latitude it allowed to suggestibility. For some the demands made upon them by a physical explanation for organic disease presented too rigid a discipline. For a time almost everything was explainable by the psycho-soma, and who could deny it? For although the soma can be identified, the psyche cannot. Was it not evident that patients with persistent diarrhoea were touchy, depressed, all too often 'off-centre'? Effect had conveniently become cause. Then in 1950 a paper was published in an American journal reporting the observation of changes in the colon which accompanied feelings of anger and hostility; this made a deep impression in gastroenterological circles, for these stressful emotions were seen to cause the mucosa to become engorged and fragile. Seeing is believing, even to psychiatrists when convenient; psychiatry had come into its own. Many were the patients whose diarrhoea was submitted to the disturbance of psychoanalysis.

Psychiatric treatment had its risks. I can recall too vividly, though it was more than thirty years ago, a nursing sister admitted under my care from a district hospital where the psychological inferences had been taken to the limit: the diarrhoea was all due to the mind. Ipso facto it only required an effort of mind, of self-discipline, to control it. Her treatment had been based upon an instruction to do so; failure was naughtiness and due to indiscipline. When incontinence ensued as it inevitably did with soiling of the bed, no immediate attempts had been made to change the soiled sheets; that was the corrective. By the time I saw her her colon had reached the stage of disintegration and her skin had broken down through persistent soiling. She died.

It was unusual for psychiatric treatment to be carried to such limits in its subservience to theory. Nevertheless it was based upon hypotheses developed from a logic peculiar to the psychiatric mind. One was the rejection-riddance theory which could be summarised thus: if you cannot stand your mother-in-law and have not the guts (sic!) to tell her so then you develop diarrhoea: the symbolic act of rejection. It became necessary to test the validity of the psychological hypotheses which began to abound. A colleague working in the same hospital with me at that time was a psychiatrist with a healthy scepticism. Every patient with ulcerative colitis seen at hospital, in my clinic or on the ward was interviewed by him and compared with a similar group with another form of gastrointestinal disturbance, usually gastric or duodenal ulcer, or gall stones. He found no evidence that psychoneurotic disorder was more prevalent in those with ulcerative colitis; however there were differences in certain particulars. There appeared to be a greater proportion of those with a sense of social responsibility, of the conscientious 'do-gooder' among the ulcerative colitic group. Moreover attacks of diarrhoea sometimes coincided with life-events such as getting engaged or married, or even more understandably, suffering grief.

Doctors working in Baltimore, USA, were unable to reveal any relationship to psychological disturbance even of this nature. But we were able to rule out the rejection–riddance theory. When undertaking each interview we took the trouble to find out what the first symptom was in each case. Because diarrhoea is the predominant feature of the disease it is often considered to be the presenting symptom, the first to become manifest. This, we found, is by no means so. In half the patients blood in the stools was the first abnormality they noticed, one which often persisted for three to four days or more before diarrhoea started, sometimes with pain which subsided as the flux followed. A condition which starts as often as not with blood in the stools could be interpreted more readily as a call for sympathy than an act of defiance or disapproval!

The scene changed; psychosomatic disorder was followed by autoimmune disease, a trend which began to obtrude on ulcerative colitis in about 1960. In a sense it was an extension of the thought that ulcerative colitis might be a manifestation of alimentary sensitivity to food in particular, a possibility which had been mooted a few decades before. Milk, suspect since the 1940s, became further incriminated by a study undertaken in Oxford in the 1960s, but only until it was realised that the adverse response to milk in sufferers from ulcerative colitis was an indication only of that small proportion of the population who have the misfortune to react to milk and its products. What this did reveal was that some of those who apparently have ulcerative colitis are in fact suffering from a food allergy, namely sensitivity to milk, the manifestations of which were previously thought to be confined to gastric reactions such as nausea and vomiting, and to skin reactions and migraine.

The excitement and hope which the Oxford reports raised, gradually subsided, but a small contribution had been made, and not only in narrowing the field as regards ulcerative colitis. For a time it had seemed possible that ulcerative colitis might be an alimentary manifestation of allergy, rather as hay fever is of an inhaled allergen. This notion was now overtaken by the concept of autoimmunity, which was more sophisticated and had arisen at that time through the discovery of the form of inflammation of the thyroid gland referred to in the last chapter, which can ultimately lead to its destruction as a functioning endocrine gland. With this thought in mind research was undertaken which led to the deduction that some individuals might develop sensitivity to elements within their own colonic mucosa, or even other structures in the intestinal wall. This possibility raised another query: why should an individual suddenly become sensitive to his own colon? Or conversely, what would make colonic tissue foreign to him, just as though it were a tissue or organ graft from someone else?

The answer came from the thyroid. It was observed that thyroiditis followed viral infections such as influenza, not always and inevitably but occasionally, in particular when associated with laryngitis; so that the nearby thyroid gland is damaged causing a leak, as it were, of thyroid material outside the confines of the gland, where it is not just unusual but abnormal and treated accordingly. Immune reactions are triggered off. Any one of the numerous viruses known to attack the gut, which have already been considered, could be responsible. Bearing in mind that it is conceivable that bacteria could achieve the same effect there is no end to the possibility of autoimmunity. This mechanism is hard to prove in the bowel if only because inflammatory reactions are a constant process within the mucosa, occurring quite properly there.

However, it was the popular thought of the 1960s that the body could develop antibodies which would destroy the epithelial cells of its own mucosa lining the bowel, through an odd quirk. The antibodies being raised by the body to protect it against the intrusion of a particular bacterium resident in the bowel, *escherichia coli*, were also found to react with the epithelium. Although later disproved, the autoimmune concept did carry the management of ulcerative colitis a stage forward by justifying treatment with steroids which act by attacking inflammation through blocking immune responses. Moreover it concentrated research upon the significance of what is going on in the mucosa and on the purpose of the inflammatory cells there, research which continues today to find out if immune processes developing within the mucosa are involved in colitis of either type, Crohn's or ulcerative. Even if the initial damage is not brought about by this means at least it seems possible that the persistence of chronicity of both ulcerative colitis and Crohn's disease could be the outcome of immunological mechanisms brought into play by whatever may have caused the gut to rot.

Thereafter investigation into the possible causes of ulcerative colitis tended to lapse as the limelight turned towards Crohn's disease, which began to obtrude more upon medical consciousness the world over as it came to be seen more often. There have been recent flickerings in the ulcerative colitic field; the age-old thoughts about a bacterial infection have been resuscitated rather indirectly, due more to developments in the microbiological field than to those in gastroenterology.

The early 1970s, which saw a special bacterium attack man for the first time in the form of Legionnaire's disease, also saw another 'new' disease, acute enteritis caused by an organism known as campylobacter. In fact the bacterium was not new to science, for it had been discovered in animals in 1913 as a cause of veterinary disease. It had not been thought to be troublesome in man for the simple reason that it had not been isolated by microbiologists from the stools of patients until 1971, when it was first found in patients in Australia followed by a similar discovery in Brussels. To demonstrate the presence of campylobacter, which is a near relative of the vibrio of cholera, it is necessary to develop a culture medium which will inhibit the other 400 odd organisms common to the gut from overwhelming it. This the veterinary bacteriologists had achieved; in the 1970s medical science began to take a leaf out of the veterinary book. Since then it has become clear that, unlike Legionnaire's disease, the diarrhoea caused by campylobacter is no new disorder. It was there all the time undetected. Moreover it is now obvious that it is the commonest cause of dysentery and, indeed, of admissions to hospital on account of diarrhoea. It seems probable that it is of even greater importance as a cause of diarrhoea in the tropics. In short, more and more is still being learnt about campylobacter and the way these organisms (for there is a family of campylobacter) affect man. We have recently discovered that, although the small bowel is the primary target, campylobacter can and does attack the colon. No doubt some patients labelled with the diagnosis of ulcerative colitis in the past have had this specific infection.

But the discovery of campylobacter raises a disquieting thought and indeed a problem. What other infections of the gut are we missing through ignorance as to how to approach them, to lure them from obscurity into open culture so that they can be seen, studied and identified? Is ulcerative colitis going to prove to be a conglomerate of as yet undetectable and so undetected infections? These uneasy thoughts were further reinforced towards the end of the 1970s by the emergence of yet another bacterium from the limbo where it had been lurking unobserved, also because of difficulty in culturing it.

The story starts with the advent of antibiotics; from their introduction with penicillin an acute form of colitis was encountered as a complication from time to time in patients receiving them. The acute colitis was not new for it had been described in the pre-antibiotic era together with the peculiarly distinctive cast of the bowel which is shed and passed in the stool when the infection takes hold. When penicillin and the powerful antimicrobial drugs like chloramphenicol and tetracycline which followed penicillin came in, it struck more frequently. Since antibiotic misuse had led to the emergence of an antibiotic resistant staphylococcus causing infections in wounds and elsewhere, this microbe was sought for in the stools of such patients, and found. From which it was not unreasonable to conclude that the staphylococcus was the nigger in the woodpile encouraged by antibiotic suppression of other organisms; a thought reinforced by the knowledge that staphylococci contaminating food from infected fingers of food handlers can produce a toxin which attacks the intestine.

139

By 1970 new forms of penicillin, clindamycin and lincomycin, had been introduced; matters took a turn for the worse; pseudomembranous colitis began to occur more frequently. A year or two earlier it had been discovered in the laboratory that hamsters developed colitis when given clindamycin and indeed that they seemed generally susceptible in this way to many antibiotics. What was more, the inflammation was not due to chemical damage brought about by the antibiotic; ten years were to elapse before a specific bacterium was found to be the cause. It turned out to be a clostridium, one of a large family resident in the gut of various animals, of which that causing tetanus in man is but one member. *Clostridium difficile* had first been isolated in 1935; it earned its name because of the difficulty experienced in culturing it and for thirty years it had remained undetected in humans for it is by its nature fastidious – microbiologists use that very word, labelling it a 'fastidious anaerobe'. In other words attempts to culture it in an atmosphere deprived of oxygen will not suffice; special attention is required in addition to encourage it to grow.

Small wonder then that *clostridium difficile* had not been isolated from human stools. In the light of the findings in hamsters renewed attempts were made in patients with antibiotic associated colitis. The presence of *clostridium difficile* was confirmed. Like all clostridia, *difficile* creates havoc through a toxin and this is easier to demonstrate in the stool than the presence of the organism. Since it, rather than the staphylococcus, has been established as the agent causing pseudomembranous colitis, the next step has been to look for it or, to be more exact, for the toxin in ulcerative colitis, because of the near impossibility of capturing the organisms in culture when they are sparsely dispersed. The result has been tantalising; the toxin is sometimes there, sometimes not. Moreover it has been discovered in patients with diarrhoea who have never received antibiotics. What is more, it is catching. Once introduced into a ward it can spread to other patients, and even across the corridor to the ward on the opposite side.

Can this be the culprit in ulcerative colitis? Probably not, since it is too contagious; ulcerative colitis can persist for years in one patient without contaminating others near by. In addition, *difficile* toxin does not show up in every case of ulcerative colitis. But the *denouement* of *clostridium difficile* has served to reinforce the feeling that our understanding of intestinal horticulture is rudimentary, and that we have a long way to go before the activities of micro-organisms, to say nothing of their presence in the gut, are fully understood. Clues to some of the mechanisms involved in ulcerative colitis may well be hidden there.

Meanwhile one further clue has come to light, a clue we can as yet make nothing of, which runs counter to received knowledge to date, and will upset the zealots of the anti-smoking lobby. It first appeared almost as an aside in a brief article in the *British Medical Journal* in 1982, almost as a curiosity, to the effect that in the health area served by Cardiff non-smokers are in greater preponderance among ulcerative colitic patients than in the population at large or in those with Crohn's disease. There followed, in subsequent weeks, some anecdotal fag ends of support in the correspondence columns followed by a flicker of support from Czechoslovakia; then the fag went out. But not for long. In 1983 came a report from Boston, USA, culled from large numbers of patients who had been under review since 1966 for other reasons; the risk to smokers of getting ulcerative colitis is less than a third compared with non-smokers. Later in that year a study from Nottingham of impeccable epidemiological standard showed this unexpected revelation to be highly significant statistically.

What can be made of this? Two possible explanations come to mind. Firstly, that it may be due to a pharmacological effect; nicotine has a direct effect on large bowel activity. As many smokers are aware, bowel movements can be induced by smoking a cigarette or a pipe. Indeed that could provide another explanation: that those with ulcerative colitis refrain from smoking so as to avoid contributing further urgency to their diarrhoea. But that implies too great a prescience; in the Nottingham series those who have never smoked contribute to the nine-fold difference in

141

susceptibility. Future patients can hardly foretell what will befall them. More plausible is the thought that ulcerative colitic patients are drawn from the more conscientious and more responsible members of society, as the psychiatrist and I found all those years ago in Birmingham, and so are less likely to take up smoking or, if they have done so, more likely to give it up. That could be put to the test if it were possible to study the population which existed before smoking became taboo. It is, however, very unlikely that a personality factor will be disposed of in this way because smoking habits were not recorded with such diligence before the lung cancer scare started and was proved. Nevertheless more will undoubtedly be heard of this. For the present all that can be said is that non-smoking appears to be an aetiological factor. And what about Government health warnings now?

*

Understandably ideas about the causation of Crohn's disease have followed much the same paths. In this they may be misleading, for one problem turns upon whether Crohn's disease is new. The ecology of man is in a state of constant change not least as regards the diseases to which he is prey. While some cancers disappear others raise an ugly head; just as smallpox is being seen off, Legionnaire's disease and lassar fever begin to make themselves felt, and even more recently, AIDS. So there is nothing strange about the proposition that Crohn's disease made its first appearance at the turn of the century. Evidence to support this lies in the fact that it was first noticed as a distinct entity by Dalziel around 1910 onwards. Crohn's ileitis could however have been so merged in tuberculous enteritis as to be indistinguishable before this so that it did not come readily to light. Yet there is another pointer to it being a new disease – the rapid increase of cases throughout the world, more particularly in recent times. This looks like a new entity getting under way. In the 1950s it was virtually unseen in Australia; it is commonplace in gastrointestinal practice there now. During the twenty years which followed, the annual number of new cases more than doubled in England and Scandinavia; in effect this was found to be so anywhere where it was possible to carry out sound epidemiological studies in stable populations without the difficulty of having to discount the possibility that the disease was being recognised for the first time.

For the moment let us take it that Crohn's disease is new. If so it could be due to change in the milieu which surrounds us. The thalidomide tragedy focussed attention sharply upon the importance of environmental factors other than infections in the making of disease. The foetus and the young child are particularly susceptible because of the increased cellular turnover and vulnerability of their cells as they are growing up.

In my student days there was an obscure weakness which affected babies up to the age of three years or so; the cause of that has now come to light. It was lead in the paint which covered the cot rails which they sucked and the toys they put in their mouths. We no longer see this lead neuropathy now that lead has been withdrawn from a baby's immediate environment. We are now proceeding to chase the lead out of petrol and replacing lead water pipes with copper ones. This may be as well for another reason, for although without a shred of evidence or a vestige of proof, lead along with mercury has been one of the innumerable substances to come under suspicion in Crohn's disease.

Suspicion that a toxic agent may be at fault is aroused when a disorder has no visible cause as obvious as a micro-organism or a parasite; it can still prove difficult to detect for the search has to be conducted on the basis of enlightened guesswork, often along devious paths. Like the nitrosamines found to be the cause of the phenomenal increase in cancer of the gullet from 1950 onwards in Bantu tribesmen. Nitrates, which form an inevitable part of our diet, can be converted to nitrites when food is preserved; the nitrites then combine with amines from alcohol fermentation in gastric juice to form nitrosamines. In addition nitrites are used as fertilisers; these compounds can accumulate in plants and vegetables where molybdenum is

143

deficient from the soil they are grown in. Molybdenum deficiency affects the soil in Transkei.

In the face of such complex mechanisms and such a host of unimaginable unknowns a long time can pass before a toxic environmental agent is pinned down; one could have eluded us in the half century since Crohn described the disease, particularly as little investigation has been concentrated upon this possibility. Considerably more effort has been expended upon looking for evidence of an infective agent; oddly, perhaps, because an infection might be expected to have made itself evident in one way or another during that time. But just as the environment presents an ever changing scene as regards the harmful chemicals we are subjected to, so the micro-organisms around us can change their habits. One manner in which this comes about is by mutation, so that a benign virus, for example, can breed almost overnight a new generation equipped through change in its nuclear materials to do harm to man.

A mutation of this kind taking place at about the turn of the century would match the way the disease has taken hold better than the impingement of a new toxic agent or some nutritional deficiency, the latter being an unlikely cause since Crohn's disease affects the developed society of the western world in preference to the third world.

A new infection would take time to build up thus accounting for the way in which the incidence of the disease has been increasing recently, particularly if the organism responsible displayed low infectivity and low penetrance, by which is meant, on the one hand the power of contagion, and on the other the ability to gain a foothold within the human frame; it might also have a long incubation period. All these characteristics would be required of any infective agent which was to account for this disease.

It was with these thoughts in mind that we started to look for a possible infective agent in about 1970 at St George's Hospital. As so often in research our initial aim had a rather different purpose: the need to find out more about how azathioprine worked. Its effect in the treatment of Crohn's disease, as related earlier, was so capricious and yet so notable when it did take effect that I decided that we should set up a model of Crohn's disease in animals to enable us to study the effects of the drug. A suitable likeness to the disease had been brought about in rabbits by Slaney, a colleague who was working in Birmingham with me in the 1950s, later to become president of the Royal College of Surgeons. He achieved the model by the simple expedient of injecting extracts of Crohn's tissue from patients into the intestinal wall of a rabbit.

At the time we were putting this in train, a report was published from the tuberculosis research unit of the Medical Research Council indicating that whatever might be the cause of Crohn's disease it looked as though it was capable of transmission into a laboratory animal, in this case the mouse. The two doctors behind this report, Mitchell and Rees, had revived a method originally used to make possible the study of the micro-organism responsible for leprosy. Leprosy is related to tuberculosis for both are brought about by mycobacteria. Likewise there are similarities in the microscopic pattern of the lesion; as would be expected, a granuloma is to be seen. *Mycobacterium leprae* has always proved difficult to grow upon culture media or in the broths ordinarily used in a bacteriological laboratory. It had at last been achieved by the device of injecting infected material from a patient into the footpad of a mouse where the organism thrived.

This may seem rather a far cry from Crohn's disease, and certainly the approach taken by Mitchell and Rees came indirectly via a condition known as sarcoidosis. Without going too closely into details of that disease it should be said that it presents many similarities to Crohn's disease. It is of recent 'origin', it is a form of chronic inflammation but not, apparently, an infection for no infective cause has been disclosed, and the hallmark of the disease as identified in affected tissue by the microscope is very like that seen in Crohn's disease – a localised granuloma which does not go the whole way and break down to produce pus which the tuberculous granuloma does. Apart from this, sarcoidosis like Crohn's disease resembles tuberculosis, more so in fact since it is commonly located in the chest causing lymph glands there to enlarge. Other sites can be involved in sarcoid change, the skin being one where the ulceration it causes looks uncommonly like what may be seen when Crohn's disease attacks the skin, which it rarely does. To cap it all sarcoidosis shows the same tendency for activity to be followed by natural remission; it almost seems to be Crohn's disease without the predilection for the gut.

The thought was that sarcoidosis could be a latent form of tuberculosis or even some form of reaction of immunity to the mycobacteria responsible for tuberculosis, lying dormant in part or in whole somewhere in the body. If so the leprosy model which had enabled another mycobacterium to come to life in the laboratory might turn up trumps again, this time for sarcoidosis. And so it did to the extent that the cellular pattern of the disease was discerned microscopically in samples taken from the footpads of mice after they had been injected there with sarcoid material taken from patients. But no bacteria were to be seen. Mitchell and Rees had, in effect, succeeded in transmitting sarcoid into an animal, thus indicating that some noxious agent was present at the site of the disease – an antigen for want of a better term.

It was a short step to undertaking the same experiment with Crohn's material. Lo and behold, lesions developed in the footpads, though after rather a long time, for it took as long as two years sometimes before they became evident on biopsy. As Mitchell and Rees claimed, this was the first real evidence that a transmissible agent might be the cause of Crohn's disease since Dr Crohn and his colleagues had postulated at the outset a variant of tuberculosis as the cause, but had failed to obtain evidence of such an infection after injecting material from their cases into guinea pigs, rabbits and chickens. Possibly they did not wait long enough to allow the disease to take hold before looking for a positive reaction; their report gives no indication in this respect.

In our experiments Crohn's tissue was injected into the small intestinal wall of a special breed of rabbit, the New

Zealand white rabbit; this was done by opening the rabbit's abdomen in an operation no less carefully conducted than any operation on a patient, and then making the injection under direct vision. Since the epidemiology of Crohn's disease in man made it clear that an infection, if that was the cause, must have a long incubation period, we resisted the urge to have a further look inside too soon, waiting for three months, a relatively long time in a rabbit's existence, before making the first inspection of the intestines; thereafter, if nothing appeared to be wrong, looking again at six and then nine months after the injections were made. We were encouraged to find appearances in every way resembling Crohn's disease: the long strictures, the multiple 'skip' lesions, the thickening of the mesentery with fat spreading from it around the affected areas; not in every animal, but in enough to make it seem significant. Moreover microscopic examination revealed not only granulomas but ulcers with a tendency to penetrate as though they might become fistulas. By this time the research fellow working with me, David Cave, and Don Mitchell had joined forces; the chase after the transmissible agent was on.

There are several ways of conducting such a chase; ours was through an endeavour to identify the features of this foreign agent. This necessitated preparing in a special way abnormal tissue obtained at an operation on a patient; injecting an extract into a batch of rabbits or mice, while at the same time injecting a similarly prepared extract of normal human intestine into other rabbits or mice for comparison; keeping all the animals alive for three, six or nine months, and operating upon them at intervals – a lengthy, tedious and expensive search. One important clue to the nature of the beast would be its size. So one experiment was undertaken using the mashed up extract of Crohn's tissue after it had passed through filters of varying size before being injected into the animals. The outcome showed the agent to be small, small enough to be a virus or possibly a bacterium capable of changing its shape and wriggling through the mesh of the finest filter. And there

147

we got stuck, unable to demonstrate visually either form of micro-organism, though we were able to transmit the agent from animal to animal and from one generation to another, up to four generations (we did not carry on beyond that).

Meanwhile others elsewhere were endeavouring to reproduce these results and obtain their own laboratory models of Crohn's disease. Some failed to do so, so were we wrong? Claim and counter-claim has ever been the course of biological research. Though the concoction of an extract of Crohn's tissue taken from an operation specimen is in principle a straightforward affair, the actual recipe is complex. It began to appear that the steps in its execution had to be followed precisely; despondency and doubts were dispelled by reports of success when this was achieved elsewhere.

In the USA the agent was being pursued on different lines. On the assumption that it might be a virus, extracts of Crohn's tissue were placed upon cell cultures. The cultures ceased to thrive, presumptive evidence that a virus was present gnawing away at the cells. Next, cell cultures were prepared from the intestinal epithelium of New Zealand white rabbits, again with positive results; then from the same source came news that with the aid of the electron microscope the virus had actually been seen lurking in the cell culture. That was in the summer of 1976; hope ran high but as time passed, it became more and more evident that it had been too fleeting a glimpse, for others could not repeat the sighting. In the surgical department at St George's Hospital where work was being continued by my successor, Hermon-Taylor, another explanation for the damaging effect of diseased tissue on cell cultures came to light; extracts taken from the inflammatory process itself rather than a micro-organism could bring about death or sickness of cells in culture. Many are the viruses which exist in normal intestine let alone an abnormal one; their identification one from another is no easy task particularly as their small size and the restriction of their composition to nuclear material without surrounding cytoplasm diminish such distinguishing marks as shape and size. Compared with a bacterium the task of establishing one particular virus as the cause of a specific disease is more difficult to achieve. So reluctantly it had to be conceded that no viral cause had yet been disclosed.

As support for a virus waned attention was suddenly drawn to a promising if obscure organism. It had the right pedigree: it was a mycobacterium, not however *tuberculosis* but *mycobacterium kansasii*. Surprisingly it was isolated in London, for as its name implies its activities are better known on the other side of the Atlantic where its attentions are usually confined to the lungs. Now *mycobacterium kansasii* had been found lurking in a lymph gland draining an area of intestine involved in Crohn's disease.

It seemed the perfect answer for more reasons than one. It would explain the granuloma accepted as the hallmark of Crohn's disease. In the USA two or three years earlier a proclivity had been observed for mycobacteria generally on the part of the lymphocytes taken from patients with Crohn's disease, those very cells, that is, which participate directly in immune responses and which take such a conspicuous part in that histological hallmark. Some twelve years earlier a young research worker in London had reported seeing with the aid of an electron microscope particles in areas affected by Crohn's disease which looked like fragments from the capsules of bacteria. Like all mycobacteria, the *kansasii* variety are wrapped in a capsule formed of fatty material, mycolic acid (hence the name *Mycobacterium*). This acid is sizeable in molecular terms so the capsule is thick relative to the rest of the rod-like bacterium. The bacteria have the ability to dismantle; by shedding their capsules they become vulnerable but more mobile. The thin flexible rod left after shedding the mycolic straight jacket can with a little distortion worm its way through a fine filter.

It began to look as though *mycobacterium kansasii* fitted the bill and fulfilled the requirements we had been looking for as a result of the experimental work indicating a transmissible agent. But it was not to be. Again hopes were dashed. No part of the mycobacterium, let alone the whole organism, could be found in diseased tissue. Nor was it possible to induce a skin reaction in patients to extracts of the organism, a reaction which should have proved positive if *mycobacterium kansasii* was the cause. The final blow came when it became obvious that it had only been found on one occasion from one gland draining a specimen removed at operation. It was never seen again, anywhere. Perhaps the urge to find a mycobacterium had become father to the thought that it had been discovered.

Possible contenders have been sought among bacteria ordinarily found in the gut, but without success. An odd little parasite, small enough to live in human cells, has been invoked if only because one form is known to provoke a rare disease located in the rectum which has some resemblance to Crohn's disease (including fistula formation), and because it can attack the intestine of cattle and sheep. The family of chlamydia came to notoriety in the 1920s when psittacosis was brought into the UK by parrots, leading to a ban in their import until recent times. A new cause for notoriety rests with *chlamydia trachomatis* which used to confine its attention to the eye but has now become one of the numerous agents in sexually transmitted disease, and a common one at that. A solitary report from Rotterdam that Crohn's patients possess antibodies against chlamydia was not so far fetched as at first it might have seemed, for when psittacosis attacks man it causes diarrhoea amongst other symptoms, and is inclined to resemble typhoid. Could there be a link between the increasing prevalence of *chlamydia trachomatis* and Crohn's disease? If so, no further support has been forthcoming for this contender.

A profusion of immune reactions have been considered: one, that repeated damage to the mucosa by bacterial forays from the gut could bring about a persistent reaction by immunological cells to the damaged epithelium: another, that the disease represents a reaction *ad infinitum* due to the presence of fragments of bacteria, killed and all but eliminated, exhausting the effectiveness of the immune response so that the reaction between the lymphocytes and the noxious agent persists through the inability to gather

150

enough immunological strength to master the intrusion and settle it once and for all.

So by fits and starts the story of the transmissible agent progressed – hardly the appropriate word, perhaps, since we seem to be no forrader. But are we back where we started? Not quite, if only because a few contenders have been crossed off the list. The real question now is whether there is a transmissible agent. This has certainly not been conclusively proved, but ask anyone working in the field their opinion – and there are now quite a few around the world: they still express their uncertain view that the cause of Crohn's disease is probably transmissible. But on that particular tack it has to be admitted that research has run into the doldrums; little that is new has turned up in the last seven years.

Attention has turned rather desultorily to nutritional factors. Again epidemiological patterns could be construed as incriminating what we eat. At the present the disease is rare in the orient and the tropics, commoner in western societies. One explanation could be in the contribution made by refined sugars and carbohydrates generally to the diet of the more developed world. Cereals came under suspicion because the breakfast bowl of cornflakes was recently found to be taken more often by Crohn's patients than others. This caused a temporary flutter at the breakfast table for it was said to be a significant finding at that particular meal but not if the cornflakes were eaten later in the day. This observation was probably a statistical quirk for it has not been confirmed elsewhere, though there had been a report from Germany a year or two earlier suggesting that those who develop Crohn's disease had eaten more pastries and sweets than those who are well.

Little confidence can be placed on reports which rely upon the recollections of patients as to what have been their eating habits going back over many years, and it is unlikely that an item of diet would be effective in the short term. Nevertheless the possibility that harm comes the intestinal way through what is eaten is real indeed and not confined to the vagaries of nutrition. In the host of additives in use –

the spreaders, the sweeteners and the preservatives – who knows what substances innocuous in themselves may lurk to become harmful in conjunction with other material or in the ever changing milieu of the intestine?

*

In conclusion, where do matters stand in respect of the nature of these two enigmatic conditions, ulcerative colitis and Crohn's disease? What will the future bring?

It appears to me possible that effort and expense may be wasted if too much time is spent pursuing a cause for ulcerative colitis, for I do not believe that this is a disease *sui generis*. Back in 1934 dysentery attacked 210 individuals in an epidemic in New Jersey caused by one of the shigellae named appropriately after a famous New York bacteriologist, Dr Flexner. These patients, or rather 122 of the 210 originally involved, were kept under surveillance; after a year ten per cent continued to have symptoms although all trace of Flexner's bacillus had disappeared. They had developed ulcerative colitis. Indeed Hurst, the father of British gastroenterology, had reported at much the same time that among his patients with ulcerative colitis were men who had contracted bacillary dysentery in the first world war, an observation repeated by others after the second war. In my own practice I have likewise treated patients for ulcerative colitis which dated from an episode of dysentery in the second world war when the diagnosis had been well established. Similarly amoebic dysentery can provide the starting point of persistent or recurrent diarrhoea continuing long after the parasite has been eliminated. It appears that if damage to the colonic mucosa is of sufficient severity it will sap its integrity to such an extent as to cause further ulceration in the future even after healing has taken place. Certainly the epithelial cells which reform and restore the surface when the ulcers heal are sometimes abnormal, being less than their proper height. They may be defective in other ways and less able to stand up to constant assaults from the tumultuous events within the bowel lumen, or less capable of preventing bacterial penetration.

The mechanism may be less obvious and direct. Damage

brought about by any of a multitude of known, identifiable and detrimental agents, mostly micro-organisms, could set going an abnormal immune complex which persists within the mucosa to become active under the mildest stress – a trigger cocked, set to go off at the lightest touch. Immune reactions within the inflamed intestine are known to be responsible for such complications of ulcerative colitis as develop elsewhere in the body – arthritis and eczema. The same mechanism may account for the peeling of the epithelial surface of the intestine just as it does the skin in cases of eczema. The harm which sets matters in train, though identifiable, may frequently pass undetected. Ulcerative colitis is no more than an abnormal state which results from the response to any blow which can beset the large intestine, though it is not an inevitable response to every ill the colon is heir to.

Crohn's disease is another matter. It does have more the appearance of a disease in its own right; it looks less like an abnormal state brought about by a variety of causes than a dynamic process set in train by a specific event and persisting long after that cause has come and gone. For Crohn's disease is not confined to an anatomical area of known predilection to certain parasites and micro-organisms. The distinctive ulceration, apart from affecting any part of the gut from top to bottom, can be seen elsewhere, in the skin for example. Crohn's disease is capable of becoming generalised in a way that ulcerative colitis is not.

Will a cause for Crohn's disease be found? Not until prevailing attitudes change, and we rid our minds of convention, one of which is general: a tendency to think in terms of a sole cause. Such is the complexity of pathological change in Crohn's disease that it appears unlikely to be the outcome of one single cause with one immediate effect. Something else goes on between the moments of initiation and revelation. There appears to be a dynamic process set in train by an initial incident, which is thereafter perpetuated by a cascade of events. So we must widen our perspective from the customary vision of one cause for a disease. We have to learn to expect an involved chain of reaction ensuing from a beginning of such apparent insignificance as hardly to merit the word cause.

The other attitude which has to change lies in the experimental approach. The use of experimental animals, the rat, the mouse, the rabbit and the guinea pig, has become inappropriate, as has that of the larger animals – cats, dogs and monkeys. Quite apart from the fact that they are too expensive to obtain and maintain, their use has become inept because of the many uncertainties of interpretation which arise. How can we be sure that the reaction seen under a microscope is not due to the trauma of innoculation rather than the effect of the innoculum? That changes seen after a long period of surveillance of a mouse should not be ascribed to ageing? To eliminate these awkward questions litter mates have to be kept for comparison, some being subjected to innoculation without the specific innoculum. At best this is expensive, at worst uncertain.

The problems are greater the other way round. When nothing happens how can we be sure that we have chosen an animal which will react like man? The imponderables of experiments using animals in the search for an unknown cause of a chronic disease are too great; the observations required have to go on for too long. Not only do such investigations become expensive; too many animals may die so that valid conclusions cannot be drawn. In summary, animal experiments for this purpose are too crude, though that is not to say that animals are not essential in other fields of research: in particular for assay and identification of recognisable culprits in the microbial field.

Our understanding of biological processes is now soundly based at the molecular level in biochemistry; it has moved to the cellular level in anatomy. The electron microscope has permitted us entry into the cell by insight into its workings, thus revealing the relationship between chemical function and structural form. It has brought in its train the greatest revolution in biological comprehension since Vesalius began to publish accurate descriptions of the structure of the human body in the sixteenth century. Electron microscopy has now been turned to the abnormal cell; it is achieving in disease what it has already done in normality, to an extent that breaks down even further the boundaries between normal and abnormal. It is now hard to know where one ends and the other begins. The solution to the problems posed by Crohn's disease will in future be found in the study at molecular level of biological fluids and cellular extracts. When a living model is required it will not be an animal but a cell, not in the form of sheets of cells in culture familiar to us today but as individual units through harvesting protozoa, large ones like amoebae, into which to inject significant extracts from the abnormal areas presented by the disease, and observing the results in molecular terms.

An understanding of terms

ACID, ACIDITY. In terms of acidity and alkalinity the *milieu interieur* of the body is neutral and has to remain so to be compatible with life. In order to maintain this neutrality water and electrolytes must remain in balance. Nevertheless fluids secreted or excreted may fluctuate widely; the juice secreted by the stomach could not be more acid; urine may be acid or alkaline. (*See also* ion and osmosis.)

AEROBE, AEROBIC. An aerobic organism requires oxygen to survive.

AETIOLOGY. A collective term for the factors contributing to disease and to the origins of diseases.

ALIMENTARY indicates a relationship to the whole of the digestive tract from beginning to end; hence alimentary tract.

ALKALINE, ALKALINITY. *See* acidity.

ALLERGEN. A substance which on contact with an individual can cause a sensitivity or allergic reaction, like pollen and hay fever. A wide range of substances are allergenic, all at points of contact – skin, respiratory system and the gut. Though similar in some respects to an antigen an allergen does not necessarily invoke an antibody reaction. The two words nevertheless tend to be used synonymously.

AMINO-ACID. Amino-acids are the basic compounds released by digestion from which whole proteins are formed and from which new proteins are built up within the body.

ANAEMIA. Essentially the state when less than the normal quantity of haemoglobin is circulating (5 g per 100 ml).

ANAEROBE, ANAEROBIC. An anaerobic organism can exist without oxygen. Some anaerobes can only exist in the absence of oxygen; facultative anaerobes are not obliged to do so.

ANASTOMOSIS. Strictly meaning a junction, the word is mostly used in a biological sense to indicate junctions brought about by operation between hollow organs such as the intestines, and blood vessels. Hollow organs are 'anastomosed'; solid structures like nerves and tendons are 'sutured'.

ANION. *See* ion.

ANTIGEN. A noxious substance which causes an immunological response. It may be a micro-organism, a toxin, a protein molecule, or a fragment of protein. Antigens bring into play antibodies specific for each antigen. Antigens usually come from the outside, but sometimes a tissue within the body or an internal secretion may become antigenic.

157

ANTIBODY. A substance formed by the immunological system of the body to counteract an antigen.

ANUS. The alimentary exit at which the main structure is a muscle permitting voluntary control over defaecation.

AUTOLYSIS is the beginning of bodily dissolution which follows death.

BACTERAEMIA. A condition where bacteria are present and circulating in the blood, contaminating though not actually infecting it. (*See* septicaemia.)

BACTERICIDAL indicates the ability to kill bacteria.

BACTERIUM. A unicellular organism of microscopic proportion containing a nucleus and cytoplasm which in contrast to a protozoon lives and hunts in packs.

BILE. Fluid excreted by the liver into the duodenum containing yellow pigments from the breakdown of haemoglobin, certain salts necessary for the emulsification of fats to enable their digestion, and other substances.

BIOPSY. A small specimen of tissue obtained for the purpose of investigation usually for microscopy though occasionally for bacteriological study.

BONE MARROW. Bones are not solid; they would be too heavy if they were. They are for the most part hollow or latticed in the centre. Advantage is taken of this space to provide an area where blood cells of all varieties can be produced.

CAECUM. The small intestine does not join with the large bowel in a direct line but from one side thus delineating a short section from the rest of the colon. This is the caecum, an area therefore distinguished by its anatomy rather than any specific function, and by the fact that the appendix gains attachment to it.

CARRIER STATE. A situation whereby a harmful micro-organism, usually a bacterium (as far as we know), can take shelter in an individual without inflicting illness upon him but can prove to be a menace to others.

CATHETER. A tube of flexible soft material, very rarely rigid, made to be passed into hollow organs, the commonest form being a urinary catheter used to empty the bladder.

CATION. *See* ion.

CELL. A cell is the basic structure of any tissue, indeed of life itself, the brick from which the body is built. A mature cell has a recognisable shape, appropriate to its place in the order of things, and a specific function. It also has a distinctive anatomy with an outer membrane containing cytoplasm, or cell sap, within which lie what are known as the organelles – structures which conduct the function of the cell. In the centre of the cell within the cytoplasm lies the nucleus containing RNA to command and control the cell's activity and DNA to ensure its perfect replication. (*See also* mutant).

CICATRISATION. The formation of scar: scarring.

CLINICAL. Pertaining to the manifestations of a disease in terms of the patient's history, symptoms and the abnormalities found on examination, which are spoken of as the signs.

CLONE. The identity of cells and the constancy of their function is a matter of continuity and is achieved by their constant replication; hence a specific line of cells, or clone, is formed to last out the time of the host. This steady state may be disturbed by mutation giving rise to a new clone.

COLON. The greater part of the large intestine, all, in fact, except the rectum.

COLOSTOMY. An artificial outlet from the colon.

CONGENITAL. From birth; usually applied to disease or malformation, which may also be hereditary.

CONNECTIVE TISSUE. What it says. Nerves and blood vessels are a form of connective tissue though the term is frequently applied to what appears to be non-descript cellular packing.

CONTROLLED TRIAL. A system applied in an attempt to achieve Cartesian standards in the immensurable fields of biology. Information is sought in the group being studied and compared with a group (the control group) alike in every way but not subject to the influence being investigated. With the assistance of statistics a positive answer is assumed from small numbers thus reducing time and numbers in clinical investigations. Perfectionists demand blind and even double blind trials, by which is indicated a random selection of individuals to each group so as to avoid bias on the part of the investigator. They also insist on statistical significance which has become a catch phrase for veracity, a parrot cry at scientific meetings.

CRYSTALLOID. A simple chemical compound or salt which will dissolve in water, so simple that the size of the particles in solution is less than one micron in diameter.

CYSTIC FIBROSIS. A congenital disease which, *inter alia*, denies pancreatic ability to secrete.

CYTOPLASM. *See* cell.

DEHYDRATION. When the body loses water it is said to be dehydrated. But in terms of its fluid component the body has three compartments – in the blood vessels, in the tissue spaces and within the cells themselves. Each compartment may be differently affected depending upon the circumstance of dehydration.

159

DIAGNOSIS. Knowing the answer as to what the disease is. There is often no simple answer. Influenza is a clinical diagnosis only; it does not indicate the causative factor. Tuberculosis does bespeak the cause but tells us no more; pulmonary tuberculosis is more informative. Diagnosis literally means to know thoroughly. So Crohn's disease can hardly be regarded as a diagnosis, only as a label for a clinical picture of disease.

DNA. *See* mutant and nucleoproteins.

DUODENUM. That part of the intestine which immediately follows the stomach. Its functions are much the same as the rest of the upper part of the small intestine, only more so. Like 'caecum' it is a street name given for location and guidance.

DYSPAREUNIA is an unnatural pain or discomfort felt by a woman on intercourse.

ECZEMA. A general term for inflammation and ulceration of the epidermis, the outermost layer of the skin. Dermatitis is a synonym. It has many causes.

ELECTROLYTE. The component parts of a salt. For example salt, per se, is sodium chloride which, on being dissolved, becomes ionised in the body to its component cation, sodium, and its anion, chloride. Electrolytes play a literally vital part in the conduct of the body's affairs in terms of water balance and the maintenance of the fine balance between acidity and alkalinity.

ELECTRON MICROSCOPE. A conventional microscope uses light waves, an electron microscope a beam of electrons with the result that it can magnify at least fifty times more than can a light microscope. The electron microscope has been able to reveal viruses to us in detail and other unthinkable minutiae, also what the fundamental working unit of the body, the cell, really looks like adding immeasurably to our understanding of how it works.

ENDOCRINE. *See* hormone.

ENDEMIC indicates continuing or recurrent infection as opposed to a limited epidemic.

ENEMA, BARIUM ENEMA. Fluid run into the large bowel per anum often for cathartic purposes but frequently to obtain an x-ray picture of the bowel using the radio-opaque material barium sulphate.

ENTERIC. Pertaining to the gut. Hence enteric fever, typhoid that is.

ENTEROCYTE. A cell belonging to the enteron, that is the intestine, often referring to the epithelial cell of the mucosa.

ENTEROTOXIC. Poisonous to the intestines.

ENZYME. An organic substance produced by a living cell which brings about a chemical or biochemical reaction without being

160

absorbed or destroyed in the process. Enzymes are essential determinants of biological reactions; a little of an enzyme goes a long way.

EPIDEMIC. An outbreak of cases of an illness.

EPIDEMIOLOGY. The study of the environmental factors which surround an illness.

EPITHELIUM. The covering layer of cells of the skin for example or the internal surface of the gut.

FAECES. Excreta from the bowel; in a word – shit.

FISTULA. An abnormal communication from a hollow organ like the gut to the skin or between loops of intestine or from one hollow organ and another.

GASTRIC. Pertaining to the stomach.

GRANULOMA. A general term given to an agglomeration of inflammatory cells.

HAEMOGLOBIN. The substance responsible for oxygen transport and delivery in the tissues, carried via the blood stream in little packets known as red blood cells.

HISTOLOGY, HISTOPATHOLOGY. The study of cells of tissues as seen under the microscope. Hence histopathology is the study of abnormal cells in the same way.

HOMOGENATE. An insoluble substance such as tissue can be minced as by a blender to very small particles which can then be suspended in solution. Homogenates are suspensions prepared all from one tissue.

HORMONE, ENDOCRINE. A hormone is a biological switch mechanism. An effector cell, often part of a ductless gland, creates a substance when necessary to turn on a target cell and make it work. An antienzyme will switch it off, if simple withdrawal of the enzyme does not do the trick. Hormones are transported by the blood. As examples: thyroxine from the thyroid has a widespread effect on the cells of numerous organs in order to raise the metabolic level at which the body is running; the numerous sex hormones have more specific effects; digestive secretions are switched on and off by hormones. The functions undertaken by hormones are almost limitless. Endocrine is a synonym for hormone.

ILEOCAECAL VALVE. A small flap valve formed by the ileum at its insertion into the large intestine.

ILEOSTOMY. An artificial outlet from the small intestine to create a false anus from the ileum on the abdominal wall.

161

ILEUM. The further half of the small intestine. There is no defined point to mark ileum from the jejunum which precedes it.

IMMUNOGLOBULIN. A complex protein material upon which antibodies are built and circulated in the blood.

INCIDENCE. The number of new cases of a condition diagnosed in a year.

IONS. Simple substances such as salt on being dissolved in water are broken down into component parts – sodium (Na) and chloride (Cl) in the case of table salt. An electric charge passed through the solution causes positively charged atoms (the cations) of sodium to be attracted to one electrode in the solution, the negative atoms of chloride (anions) to pass to the other. Sodium is the main cation in the tissue fluid enabling many biochemical reactions and processes to take place, potassium is the equivalent within the cell. Depletion of either is likely to disturb the acid/alkaline (base) balance in the body since the hydrogen ion is their only substitute and it will swing the milieu towards acidity. Likewise the chloride anion may under certain circumstances be replaced by a bicarbonate radical so turning the balance towards alkalinity. Hence the importance of preserving electrolyte balance – a difficult task with the considerable loss of simple electrolytes in diarrhoeic stools. (*See also* molecule.)

ISCHAEMIA/IC. The state when tissue, organ or limb is deprived of blood.

JEJUNUM. The upper part of the small intestine adjoining the duodenum and the ileum, responsible for the greater part of digestion.

LESION. A general term for an abnormality, often for a specific abnormality. So someone may have a lesion, the disease being unspecified, or may be said to have a tuberculous lesion which would bring a definite picture to the mind's eye.

LIVER. Its main function is to put to good purpose the products of digestion of protein, fat and carbohydrate, with some others in addition.

LUMEN, LUMINAL. The central canal of a tube is its lumen, so the gut has its luminal surface as does a blood vessel.

LYMPHOCYTE. One of the white cells of the blood, produced by lymph glands, responsible for cellular immunity.

MESENTERY. The folds of peritoneum which tether the intestine within the abdomen to the posterior abdominal wall. All communication with the intestine – vascular, nervous and lymphatic – pass to the gut within the mesentery.

METABOLIC, METABOLISM. Metabolism is a compendium word to cover every aspect of the chemical processes involved in the handling of the basic elements of food, protein, fat and carbohydrate, from the moment of ingestion through digestion to utilisation.

MICRO-ORGANISM. A small living particle visible only by magnification through a microscope. The term includes bacteria and viruses for either of which it can be used as a synonym, albeit imprecisely.

MOLECULE. The basic component in chemical terms of any substance is a molecule which is made up of atoms of a variable number of elements held together by the strong electrical charges inherent in the electrons which in their turn create the atoms. In chemical compounds the atoms of elements are parcelled into radicals which form the components of the molecule, the ions; for example the bicarbonate radical is formed from atoms of hydrogen, carbon and oxygen which hold together and present a unity under ionisation. Once a molecule is altered or broken the substance of which it was the basic particle ceases to exist as such. It has been degraded to other substances.

MORBID ANATOMY. The science and study of abnormal tissues.

MOTION. When associated with the indefinite article a motion refers to what is passed when the bowels are evacuated.

MUCOSA. The tissue lining the inner surface of the alimentary tract which conducts functions as widely diverse as the control of digestion and the conferment of immunity. Its enzymes, hormones, secretions and immunological functions render the mucosa ceaselessly active. The intestinal mucosa is a power-house of the first importance somewhat neglected as such by biologists and those who teach the young.

MUCUS. The lubricant which the body provides in various forms applicable to the sites where it is needed. It is a variable and complex chemical, a glyco-protein – that is a conjunction of sugars and proteins – which also protects mucous surfaces and probably has other functions as yet unknown.

MUSCULARIS MUCOSAE. A thin layer of muscle embedded within the intestinal wall, the contractions of which crinkle the mucosa overlying it.

MUTANT, MUTATION. A mutation is a structural or functional change in an organism which is carried forward into subsequent generations. Its heredibility indicates that the genetic coding material DNA (*see* cell) has been altered. The outcome of such change is a mutant.

163

NUCLEOPROTEINS, DNA, RNA. For an organ or tissue to survive its constituent cells need to be able to replace themselves to overcome loss due to wear, tear and ageing. This ability, together with its function, is ordained and controlled by the nucleus of each cell. The nucleoproteins therefore fall into two categories; those in combination with desoxyribonucleic acid (DNA) which provide the template for cell replication, and those combined with ribonucleic acid (RNA) which dictate cell function.

NUCLEUS. *See* cell.

OEDEMA, OEDEMATOUS. Oedema is an abnormal collection of fluid which may occur under varying circumstances of disease. In heart failure the dependent parts become oedematous; when albumin, the protein circulating in the blood, becomes depleted as a result of severe diarrhoea, oedema is less noticeable but more generalised (*see also* osmosis.).

ORGANIC DISEASE is brought about by a recognisable and identifiable cause in contrast to functional disorder which is imposed by the mind.

OSMOSIS, OSMOTIC. Salts in solution will cause water to diffuse through a semi-permeable membrane so as to equalise the molecular concentration of the solutes on either side of the membrane. Larger molecules like those of albumin will not pass through the crevices of the membrane and so will by osmosis attract water through but not drain away themselves. Thus a steady or constant state as regards water is maintained in normal tissues allowing electrolytes to move through the semipermeable membranes presented by the cell walls. Loss of albumin from the blood stream, as in diarrhoea, causes fluid to collect in the space between the cells and the blood vessels; the albumin cannot move from that space across the blood vessel wall into its lumen to restore albumin loss there.

PALLIATION. To relieve symptoms.

PANCREAS/PANCREATIN. The gland known to gourmets as the sweetbreads, responsible for the secretion of the enzyme pancreatin which digests proteins, but also for the secretion of the hormone insulin which regulates the utilisation of sugar, our principle fuel.

PATHOGEN. Any substance living like a micro-organism, or otherwise like a chemical, which causes abnormality.

PATHOLOGY. The study and science of abnormality in all its aspects though the study of abnormal tissues, as by a histopathologist, is usually what is inferred. But there are chemical pathologists, though strictly they should be called biochemical

164

pathologists; and the haematologist who is the expert in blood and its disorders is in effect a haemopathologist.

PENETRANCE. It is more a concept than a demonstrable reality that the power of a micro-organism to invade is variable and quantifiable as penetrance.

PERINEUM. That area vulgarly known as the crutch surrounding the anus, and the vagina in women.

PERISTALSIS. Gastric and intestinal movements in their various forms to impart backwards and forward and churning motion to assist mixing, digestion and absorption of their contents, and to achieve their forward progression.

PHLEGMON, PHLEGMONOUS. An archaic term for a mass of inflammation, still useful since it indicates a conglomerate of organs involved in an area of inflammation.

PHTHISIS. Pulmonary tuberculosis.

PHYSIOLOGY. The study of bodily function. One of the great nineteenth and early twentieth century biological sciences it has now served its purpose and is virtually extinct having been overtaken by the progeny it has spawned like biochemistry which in its turn has suffered a similar fate. The word retains a late twentieth century meaning and is used in a general sense to indicate the workings of a biological system.

PLASMID. A small independent particle of genetic material which may be acquired by bacteria to their advantage. It is through the acquisition of a plasmid that bacteria can obtain a shield of resistance against antibiotic attack which can be passed to future generations. Not unlike Tolkien's ring, and like that ring plasmid protection can be lost.

PREVALENCE. The number of cases of a disease known to be in existence at any one time expressed per 100,000 of the population.

PROCTOLOGIST. An expert in disease of the anus. This is so limited a field that many proctologists extend their interest to the rectum as well. The specialty has little appeal in the UK for either patients or doctors.

PROPHYLAXIS. Treatment designed to prevent a disease occurring. Vaccination is an obvious example of prophylaxis.

PROTOZOA. Unicellular organisms capable of independent existence, some of which, like the malarial parasite or *entamoeba histolitica*, achieve this at our expense.

RECRUDESCENCE. A synonym for a recurrence. Both recrudescence and recurrence imply pre-existing normality or at least a symptom-free period. A relapse may be used in this sense but it can also indicate a worsening.

RECTUM. The last part of the large bowel, with the special function of preparing for and participating in evacuation of the bowel.

REMISSION. A period of recovery.

RESECTION. Operative removal of a segment of intestine after which the open ends above and below are joined together.

SENSITIVITY. In its special medical sense this indicates an allergic response.

SEPTICAEMIA. Infection of the blood itself by live multiplying bacteria.

SERPIGINOUS. A descriptive term indicating an appearance of wandering almost exclusively used in relation to ulcers.

SERUM. The fluid part of the blood though purists would have this to be plasma and reserve the term serum for the fluid exuded from blood after it has clotted. The two have become interchangeable.

SIGMOID. The loop of large intestine between the descending colon and the rectum. Otherwise known as the pelvic colon for it hangs down into the pelvis in front of the rectum.

STEATORRHOEA. Fatty diarrhoea.

STOMA. Literally a mouth, but the word is commonly used to indicate an artificial orifice usually of an excretory nature; hence colostomy, ileostomy and urostomy.

STOMACH (GASTRIC) is not a synonym for the abdomen as so often in common parlance. It is the large receptacle which receives food from the gullet and begins to prepare it for digestion.

STOOL. Whereas a motion indicates the act of opening the bowel, the stool is the result of that act.

STROMA. That non-descript area in a tissue or organ which is best regarded as packing or framework supporting the main structure.

SUBMUCOSA. The area of ducting where nerves, vessels and lymphatics pass to and from the mucosa they serve.

SYMPTOMS are what ails the patients as opposed to signs which are the abnormalities observed in a patient.

TOXIN. Simply a poison.

THYROID. An endocrine gland in the neck which sets the level of metabolism – how high or low the flame burns.

TUBERCULOSIS. A chronic infection by mycobacteria one of which is passed from man to man, another comes through cows milk and a rare third from birds.

UROLOGY. The specialty which deals with the urinary tract.

166

VASCULAR. Pertaining to vessels – usually blood vessels.

VILLUS. The mucosa in the duodenum and a little beyond is raised into fronds; these villi provide a carpet with a thickish pile, so that more secretory and digestive cells are packed into a limited area and the absorptive surface is increased.

VIRULENCE indicates the severity of an infection and implies great potency in the organisms responsible, although the response of the host must play a part.

VIRUS. A member of that body of micro-organisms too small to be seen through a conventional light microscope and capable of passing through filters which hold back bacteria.

VITAMIN. A substance present in food in small quantities, essential to life although of no calorific value. Vitamins are catalysts in metabolic processes but cannot be synthesised in the body.

Index

abscesses: in Crohn's disease 80–1, 118, 121, 126; in ulcerative colitis 56, 57, 64–5
aetiology 133–4
amoebiasis 58–9
alcohol, effects of 32
anaemia: in cancer 91; in Crohn's disease 116; in ulcerative colitis 67, 91
anastomosis 108
antibiotics 37, 39, 40, 51–2, 99, 101–2; effects of 139–40
appendicostomy 104
arthritis, in ulcerative colitis 71
autoimmune disease 123, 136–8

bacteria: intestinal 26–7, 36–7; and toxins 36
bags: for external fistulas 84, 106–7, 108
Bargen, Dr 13, 101, 134
bed rest 120–2
Berg, surgeon 12, 13, 14
bowel movement 28
bowel surgery 103–15; aftercare 110–15
British Society of Gastroenterology 15

campylobacter 19, 138–9; jejuni 17
cancer 90–2; and Crohn's disease 86–7; symptoms 91; and ulcerative colitis 71–3
carrier infection 41–2
Cave, David 147
cells 89: inflammatory 53–6; function 54–5; malignant 90; self-replication 89

children: Crohn's disease 77–8, 88–9, 128–9; salmonella 44–5
chlamydia trachomatis 150
chocolate, salmonella in 45–6
cholera 16, 21, 29, 50; treatment 99–100
clostridium: botulinum 49; difficile 140–1
coeliac disease 30–2
colitis 53: acute 139; ischaemic 93–4; specific 50, 51; ulcerative, see ulcerative colitis
colostomy 104–6, 110
Colostomy Welfare Group 113
connective tissue 53–4
cornflakes, and Crohn's disease 151
corticosteroids 102
Crohn, Burrill 12–13, 14, 74, 77, 92
Crohn's disease 13, 15, 74–89, 92, 153–5; and acute ileitis 92; and age 74; bed rest in 120–2; cause 17, 74, 120, 138, 142–52, 153–5; as chain reaction 153–4; complications of 86–7, 126–8; diagnosis 75–7, 78–9, 129; diarrhoea in 15, 19, 74, 121, 122; location 13, 20, 74, 75, 77, 118; medical treatment 122–5; as new disease 142–3; nutrition 121–2, 151–2; progression 79–80, 85–6; recurrence 117–18, 129; and social stress 87–9; surgery 115, 116–19, 125–9;

169